Betrayal

Military trust lost as a victim of MST a teenager entering the military

George Cortez Johnson

TABLE OF CONTENTS

Preface

There is a silence that hangs thick in the air whenever the words military and trauma are paired, especially when that trauma bears the deeply personal and often invisible scars of sexual violence. For many, the military conjures images of honor, bravery, and unyielding camaraderie—a brotherhood forged in discipline and shared sacrifice. For others, especially those who enter its ranks seeking refuge from a world riddled with pain and injustice, the military holds the fragile promise of escape, stability, and a future that might outshine a troubled past. Yet, lurking beneath the rigid precision of drill sergeants and the stoic facades of service members is an undercurrent of betrayal, a hidden wound that too many bear alone: Military Sexual Trauma. This book is born from the toll of that silence, and it is a refuse pile of broken promises, but also a beacon of hope that light might still penetrate the darkness.

Betrayal tells a story that is both harrowingly specific and heartbreakingly universal. It is the story of a young African American boy who, like many young souls before him and many after, chose the military not out of sheer patriotism or simple convenience, but as a lifeline—a beacon amidst a swirling storm of gang violence, poverty, systemic racism, and the devastating crack epidemic that ravaged his neighborhood and his family. This young man stepped through the gates of the military with dreams tinted by hope, clutching tightly to the belief that here was a place where he could be more than the sum of the hardships he escaped. Instead, he found himself violently uprooted again, this time inside an institution meant to protect and empower, his body and spirit invaded by men who cloaked their hatred in the uniforms they wore and the hateful insignia they bore— men who belonged not only to the military but to the KKK, a terrifying echo of the racial hatred that stalked the streets he fled.

This betrayal is at the heart of the narrative—and it is not simply a crime against one young man's body but a brutal illustration of how the intersections of race, power, and systemic failure magnify the wounds inflicted by sexual violence. It exposes the festering rot where white supremacy and institutional repression collide, unearthing uncomfortable truths about who is vulnerable within the military's ranks and how loyalties can fracture beneath the guise of unity. The assault itself is unspeakably brutal: four white men, emboldened by their own warped sense of superiority and armed with dread threats aimed at silencing the victim through terror for his family, turn a place of potential renewal into a prison of shame and fear. Their violence does not end in that moment; it reverberates through decades, shaping the trajectory of a life in ways that ripple outward, touching relationships, self-worth, and the elusive search for peace.

But in Betrayal, trauma is not the final chapter; it is the brutal chorus that frames a story of survival, struggle, and ultimately, healing. The journey from the depths of addiction and homelessness, from fractured ties and endless nights of isolation, to the tentative hope sparked within the Veterans Affairs system reveals a path out of the shadows. The introduction to Cognitive Processing Therapy—a carefully structured mental health intervention—and the companionship of a compassionate therapist mark the beginning of reclamation. In these pages, readers will find that recovery is not linear or neat; it's messy, filled with setbacks and breakthroughs, pain and resilience. This story illuminates how validated support and understanding can plant the seeds for rebuilding trust in others and, crucially, in oneself.

Writing this book demanded a delicate balance: honoring the raw, often harsh realities of trauma and racism without succumbing to despair, while also planting the firm roots of hope and empowerment. This balance, I believe, is essential. The story is told with candor—unflinching and deeply personal—but it is also woven with moments of reflection and insight that invite readers not only to witness suffering but to grapple with its broader social context and systemic underpinnings. The narrative moves beyond the individual and into the collective, calling attention to the pervasive nature of Military Sexual Trauma and how racial dynamics and institutional culture intersect to perpetuate silence and harm.

Betrayal is first and foremost a testimony—a declaration that survivors' stories must be heard, their voices amplified, and their pain no longer dismissed or hidden behind bureaucratic walls. It is a call to action for systemic reform within the military and its veteran support systems, urging institutions to dismantle the barriers that perpetuate distrust and trauma. It seeks not only to awaken empathy but to galvanize change, fostering environments where all who serve can feel safe, respected, and truly supported. The book is also a tribute to every survivor who has endured the unbearable, suffered in silence, or struggled to be seen as more than a trauma statistic.

As you read these pages, you may find yourself sitting in uncomfortable spaces—confronting brutal truths, wrestling with emotions that range from sorrow to anger, shock to hope. You may encounter language and images that unsettle and provoke—but that is intentional. To confront these realities without flinching is a necessary step toward understanding the depth and complexity of Military Sexual Trauma, especially when it intersects with the corrosive forces of racism and hate. My hope is that you will come away not only with a deeper awareness of this issue, but also with renewed compassion for survivors and a commitment to stand alongside them.

This book does not claim to have all the answers. Recovery from such profound betrayal is ongoing and deeply personal. Yet, by sharing this story—with all its darkness and resilience—I invite readers into a conversation that has been long overdue. We must break the silence that shrouds MST, especially as it affects Black service members and marginalized communities within the military. We must dismantle the stigmas that isolate survivors and impede healing. We must advocate for justice and systemic change with urgency and fierce empathy.

If you are a survivor, a family member touched by someone's pain, a military veteran striving to carry your own struggles forward, or simply a reader who believes in the power of truth and transformation, I welcome you into these pages. May the story contained here serve as a mirror and a lamp—reflecting harsh realities and illuminating paths to healing. May it remind you that even in the face of unimaginable betrayal, the human spirit can endure, reclaim, and rise.

Together, through understanding and acknowledgement, we can help rewrite this narrative—one of courage, recovery, and unwavering hope.

George Cortez Johnson June 2024

Chapter 1
Escaping the Streets

Life in the Neighborhood

The neighborhood where I grew up was a world unto itself—an unforgiving landscape etched with the heavy marks of struggle, neglect, and a deep-seated hunger for something better that seemed to drift just beyond reach. It was one of those places that had long surrendered to cycles of poverty and violence, yet beneath the surface lay a pulse of resilience and a quiet determination from those who refused to be defined solely by their circumstances. Every day was a balance between surviving and dreaming, a tightrope walk stretched dangerously over the chasms carved out by systemic racism, gang influence, and the suffocating weight of historical disenfranchisement.

The streets we called home were marked by cracked sidewalks littered with remnants of a broken past—discarded bottles, torn posters, faded graffiti that told stories of lost hopes and battles fought silently. On the corners, groups of young men congregated, their faces hardened by experience, their eyes a complicated mix of defiance and desperation. These were places where hope and fear danced uncomfortably close, a dangerous intimacy shaped by the presence of gangs that had taken root as both protectors and predators, their flags painted not just on walls but stitched into the fabric of everyday life. Gang allegiance was almost unavoidable for many—it spanned generations, a legacy woven into the very identity of the neighborhood. It was as if survival often meant belonging to something bigger than oneself, even if that something came with the threat of violence and loss.

Gang life was not a choice in the way most people understood it—it was a gravity that pulled at you, threatening to consume any flicker of innocence or ambition before it could take flight. The pressure to conform was relentless; refusal meant isolation or worse. It was a tangled web of loyalty and fear, respect bought with blood and broken dreams. The trauma of witnessing friends caught in cycles of revenge killings or disappearing behind bars was as commonplace as breathing. I saw fathers and uncles fall victim to rivalries or police crackdowns, mothers silently mourning, their grief hidden beneath stoic faces hardened by years of pain. The crack epidemic had ravaged our community like a relentless storm; it wasn't just the drug itself but the way it tore families apart, destroyed futures, and left a trail of shattered childhoods. Kids younger than me were already shackled by addiction, their potential stolen before it had a chance to bloom.

Poverty was the soil in which all these hardships rooted themselves, its harshness unrelenting and inescapable. My own family struggled to put food on the table, often juggling multiple jobs with no benefits, no security. The city's neglect was glaring—schools were underfunded, streets remained forgotten by public works, and healthcare was a luxury rather than a right. There was an invisible divide between our world and the world just a few miles away, marked by conditions so starkly different you would think we lived in separate countries rather than the same city. Racism seeped into every crevice of life, an unseen but palpable presence that shaped interactions, opportunities, and expectations. Our faces, our accents, our very bodies seemed to echo stereotypes that others clung to tightly, using them as justifications to deny us fairness and dignity. Even authority figures who were supposed to protect us often cast suspicious glances, their biases coloring enforcement with an unfair hand.

The education system was another battlefield—classrooms that were overcrowded, teachers underpaid and overwhelmed, and textbooks several years out of date. Despite the tireless efforts of some dedicated educators, the odds felt stacked impossibly against us. Many of my peers drifted away from school, lured by the false promises of quick money and recognition offered on street corners and in back alleys. The temptation to join the ranks of those "running the neighborhood" was powerful, a seductive alternative to the daily grind of disappointment and blocked dreams. I was no stranger to the pull; I saw friends fall prey to it, their laughter replaced with guarded silence or angry outbursts, their futures dimmed before they even had a chance to define them.

Growing up, I was constantly navigating a minefield of dangers that most kids my age didn't understand. Walking home from school meant weaving through lines of drug dealers or avoiding gang territories marked by subtle but unmistakable signs—an unspoken code we all learned to read instinctively. There were nights when the distant echoes of gunfire pierced the air, rattling the thin walls of our homes and disrupting what little peace we found. In every conversation, there were whispered warnings, tales of betrayal—who to trust and who to avoid, a constant underground current of suspicion fueled by the fear that anyone could be an informant or a threat. The pressure to stay silent in the face of injustice was suffocating; speaking up risked making you a target, but silence corroded the soul with guilt and helplessness.

Amidst this harsh reality, the longing for escape grew stronger with every passing day. I watched as dreams died quietly around me— friends dropping out of school, succumbing to addiction, or disappearing behind bars. I wanted out, not just physically but mentally and emotionally. The military emerged as a beacon of hope, a promise of structure, order, and a chance to break free from the relentless grip of my environment. It wasn't just about escaping poverty; it was about carving a new identity, one that wasn't bound by the limits imposed on me by birth or place. Enlistment was painted in my mind as a pathway to stability, respect, and opportunity—an avenue to prove myself beyond the shadows cast by my neighborhood.

The decision to join the military was influenced not only by a desire to flee but also by a deep-seated hope for transformation. The media often framed the military as a meritocratic institution in which hard work and dedication could lead to upward mobility regardless of background. For someone like me, raised in the turbulence of systemic neglect and racial prejudice, that narrative was both compelling and seductive. I saw it as a chance to rewrite my story, to step into a world governed by rules rather than chaos, and to build something lasting for myself and the family I hoped to support. The thought of wearing a uniform, standing tall with a sense of purpose and belonging, offered a dream that contrasted sharply with the fractured realities I left behind.

Yet, even as I began preparing for this new chapter, the specter of my community's challenges lingered. I knew that the chains of poverty and racism didn't simply vanish with a change of address or a different role to play. The neighborhood was etched into my identity—it was the crucible that forged my resilience, even as it threatened to destroy me. The faces of those I left behind haunted my thoughts, friends caught in cycles I hoped to escape, families still struggling under the weight of systemic injustice. These contradictions fueled both my urgency to leave and my fear of what might come next. Would the military be the sanctuary I imagined, or just another battleground cloaked in a different uniform?

Amid the backdrop of urban decay and social turmoil, my inner life became a battlefield itself. The hope I clung to was fragile, vulnerable to the slightest shock or disappointment. The streets that nurtured my anger and fear also gave birth to a simmering determination. I was painfully aware of the stakes—failure wasn't just personal, it was hereditary, a curse passed down that I was desperate to break. I carried the weight of expectations from those who believed in me, and the silent judgment of those who thought I was destined to fall in line with the grim scripts written for boys born into neighborhoods like mine. This dual pressure tightened around me, making the allure of the military's promise even more potent as a lifeline, a chance to harness my spirit and rewrite my future.

In those moments of quiet reflection, I often thought about the paradoxes defining my world—the beauty and brutality intertwined with the blue skies above cracked sidewalks, the laughter mixed with sorrow echoing from stoops and worn-out playgrounds. I understood that my story was not unique but part of a larger narrative about communities pushed to the margins, about youth navigating impossible choices, about a country failing to protect its most vulnerable. This awareness sharpened my resolve to survive and thrive, even when the odds seemed daunting. The military represented the possibility of a new chapter—but little did I know that this path, too, would bring its own trials and betrayals. The journey I was about to undertake would test every ounce of that resilience born from hardship, forcing me to confront pain and courage in ways I could never have imagined.

As the day of my enlistment approached, I carried both hope and trepidation, a suitcase packed not only with clothes but with memories of a neighborhood that had shaped me in ways I was still coming to understand. Those cracked streets, the harsh lessons learned at broken tables, the faces of friends lost and families struggling—all of it was stitched into the fabric of who I was. I stepped toward the military with the dream of escape burning fiercely inside, unaware of the darkness lurking ahead, of the betrayal that would threaten to shatter not only my body but the fragile trust I held in what it meant to serve and protect. This was the beginning of a story marked by loss and recovery, by heartbreak and hope—an unflinching journey through pain toward a fragile peace.

The Crack Epidemic's Grip

In the shattered light of streetlamps, the neighborhood lay cloaked in a somber haze, a haze born not of fog but of smoke—the acrid, suffocating smoke that carried the invisible poison of crack cocaine. The epidemic had settled like an uninvited specter over every block, every stoop, and every broken fence, consuming lives with ruthless indifference. It was not just a wave of addiction; it was a tidal force that dismantled families, fractured friendships, and corroded the fragile stability of communities like the one I called home. Growing up amid the crack epidemic was akin to living under a perpetual storm cloud— thick with dread, unpredictability, and the ceaseless strain of survival.

My family, like so many others in our neighborhood, bore the weight of this plague in ways that could not easily be undone or forgotten. My mother worked tirelessly, juggling multiple cleaning jobs and an occasional shift at a diner to keep the lights on and food on the table. Yet, despite her relentless efforts, the harsh economic realities meant that the insidious reach of crack poverty gnawed relentlessly at the edges of our existence. Her exhaustion was a quiet storm; beneath her stern resolve lay a gravitational pull of worry and sorrow that she never voiced aloud but which always settled over the house like a thick quilt. The crack epidemic was the unspoken adversary in our lives, a phantom menace whose effects were etched deeply into the fabric of our daily reality.

My uncle, once a promising musician with a soulful tenor that could fill any room, had fallen victim early to the seductive grip of the drug. I remembered him from my childhood as a man of laughter and light, but by the time I was a teenager, he had become a shadow of himself, lost in a haze of desperation and fleeting highs. He moved through our home with broken eyes and trembling hands, an unsteady figure whose presence was a silent testament to the devastating toll of addiction. Family gatherings, once vibrant and filled with the harmonies of kinship and shared heritage, had been rendered fragile and sparse, held together by the moments when hope seemed not entirely extinguished. Yet, even these moments were punctuated by absences—unanswered calls, missed birthdays, and a string of hospital visits that whispered of overdose, of relapses, and of endless struggles.

Around the corner, and just across the street, my friends were caught in the same violent undertow. The innocence that should have cradled our adolescence was stolen piece by piece, replaced with the relentless pressure to survive in a landscape dominated by dealers, addicts, and an unyielding police presence that offered little protection and even less hope. In school, the desks and hallways echoed with stories of classmates who disappeared overnight, only to resurface weeks later, gaunt and hollow-eyed, or never return at all. The crime that swelled in the wake of the crack epidemic was like a beast prowling the streets, feeding on vulnerability disguised as opportunity, dragging whole generations into cycles of violence and despair.

The epidemic's influence corrupted the very notion of security within our neighborhood. Home was no longer a sanctuary but a fragile bastion against a storm that roared relentlessly outside. Fires sparked in abandoned buildings were not just accidental; they were signals of territorial fights, warnings to rivals, or funerals for lost dreams. Gunshots became a soundtrack, not an extraordinary event. Families like mine, already struggling to navigate the constant pressures of systemic poverty and racial marginalization, found themselves in impossible positions, forced to make agonizing decisions that so often had no right choices. Watching my mother grapple with those choices—balancing love, survival, and the constant threat of loss—etched a profound understanding of the suffocating limitations imposed by that time and place.

The crack epidemic was more than a socioeconomic crisis; it was a weapon wielded against communities like mine. Racist policies and neglected urban infrastructure compounded its lethality, as if the epidemic itself were a symptom of deeper systemic failures designed to push Black neighborhoods into the shadows. We bore the burden of neglect—schools starved of resources, health care insufficient for our needs, jobs scarce beyond menial labor—all while the epidemic thrived in the spaces where hope should have flourished. Every corner held stories of stolen futures, and every adult seemed haunted by the ghosts of opportunities lost to addiction and despair.

In my own heart, the epidemic swallowed my youthful dreams in moments when I confronted its reality head-on. I saw friends disappear into the maelstrom, young men who once spoke of college and music and love who instead found themselves shackled by addiction or swept into the underworld of crime and violence. The temptations were everywhere, whispers of quick money to escape the constant grind, the siren calls promising relief from the crushing burden of inequality and fear. At times, I felt the pull myself, the shadow of defeat creeping close, threatening to pull me under. But a part of me—a stubborn ember—burned with the urgent need to break free, to escape the cycle that had ensnared so many around me and that threatened to consume my very being.

This yearning to escape was not born from a single moment but from the cumulative weight of daily reality. Each time I looked around and saw my neighborhood bleeding, each time I heard the wails of sirens or the muffled cries from next door, I felt the impossible squeeze of suffocation tighten. The military emerged in my mind as more than just a job or a calling—it became a beacon of hope, a symbol of order amidst chaos, a chance at something beyond the crushing limitations of my environment. The disciplined structure, the promise of education, the escape from neighborhood violence, and the looming threats that accompanied the epidemic—these became my aspirations, my fragile lifeline.

Joining the military was, in my eyes, not only a path to stability but a rebuke to the despair that tried to claim me and those I loved. I imagined it as a clean break, a fresh chapter where identity could be rewritten beyond the circumstances of birth and environment. I dreamed of camaraderie and respect, of finding a brotherhood that valued honor over fear, strength over survival, and moral clarity over moral decay. It was not naïve to believe in that vision; it was necessary. The pain of watching my family and friends succumb to the epidemic created a void so wide and so deep that hope became an act of defiance, a rebellious streak of light standing against the darkness that threatened to consume everything.

Yet, even as I prepared to leave, the epidemic's shadow loomed large, an unrelenting reminder of the stakes involved. My mother's tearful goodbye was burdened with unspoken fears—fears of my safety in a world I could only partially understand and eyes that silently echoed the losses she had already endured. My uncle's quiet nod carried a weight of unyielding pain and perhaps a silent blessing intertwined with resignation. The friends who remained behind were caught in the inexorable tide, caught between the forces threatening to drag them under and the fragile hope that someday, somehow, they too might escape.

The crack epidemic was more than a backdrop; it was the crucible within which my resolve was forged. It was the source of my desperation and my determination—to reclaim a life stolen by circumstance. It was the reason I sought the military's promise, even if that promise, like the flickering streetlights of my neighborhood, held shadows beneath its glow. Walking away was not a simple act but a courageous leap into the unknown, propelled by every fractured memory, every lost dream, and every break of dawn I longed to see beyond the smoke.

In that grip of the epidemic's relentless hold, I found a seed of resilience, sown within the ashes of despair—a seed I nurtured quietly as I stepped forward, carrying the heavy burden of my past yet also the fragile hope of a future redeemed. The crack epidemic had claimed much of the world I knew, but it had not yet claimed me, and that small truth became the cornerstone of a journey that would test every ounce of my strength and spirit in ways I could never have imagined.

Decision to Enlist

The decision to enlist in the military was not born from naivety or youthful whimsy but stemmed from a place of deep necessity and desperation—a calculated leap into an abyss of uncertainty, fueled by the harsh realities of a life too heavy to bear any longer. Growing up in the fractured landscape of an underserved, predominantly African American neighborhood, I had long been caught in the crossfire of societal neglect, systemic racism, and the unchecked violence that choked the community like a smothering fog. The crack epidemic had gripped the streets with ruthless efficiency for as long as I could remember, carving deep wounds into families, leaving behind shattered homes and broken dreams. Gangs held dominion over corners and alleys, their unwritten rules enforced with violence that turned childhoods into grinding struggles for survival. The sirens that screamed in the night, the distant sounds of gunfire, the sorrow behind every face—these were the daily refrains echoing through my life, lessons etched into my being by the cruel hand of circumstance.

From a young age, I understood that this environment was both my prison and my battleground. Poverty strangled possibilities, suffocating any faint glimmers of hope that dared to flicker. School was more than a place of learning; it was a temporary horizon, a fragile escape from the chaos outside. But even there, the shadows of despair stretched their long fingers—underfunded classrooms, overworked teachers, and a systemic disinterest that whispered a cruel truth: I was invisible to the broader world. The dreams I nurtured, cautious and tentative as they were, found little fertile ground to grow. The rules of the streets made promises of belonging but exacted a terrible toll, and the parallel society of gang allegiances and drug trade was always lurking, waiting to pull me under its relentless current.

Against this bleak backdrop, the military began to appear as a distant beacon—a symbol of order, opportunity, and a pathway out. It represented a world where discipline could replace chaos, structure could supplant uncertainty, and where a young Black kid from the margins could forge a future untethered by the chains of his origin. I remember staring at recruitment posters plastered across rundown bus stops, glossy images of strong, uniformed figures standing proud against backdrops of freedom and duty, their smiles promising something I yearned to believe: that my life could take on meaning far beyond the narrow confines of my block. Enlistment became not just a choice but a calculated escape hatch, a way to rewrite the narrative writ in the scarred streets of my hometown.

The thought process was complex and deeply conflicted. There was fear and skepticism, of course; I wasn't blind to the stories of those who had gone before me, stories whispered in cautious tones about the military's brutal demands and the unspoken code of silence that shrouded its darker corners. But overshadowing that was a fierce hunger for transformation—a determination to break free from poverty's relentless grip, to escape the suffocating presence of gangs and drugs, and to carve a place in a world that often seemed indifferent to my very existence. The military promised a fresh start, an identity unburdened by racial prejudice or neighborhood affiliations, at least on the surface. It offered training, education, a steady paycheck, and the chance to serve something greater than myself. In many ways, it was the rare institution that seemed to extend an invitation—albeit fraught with its own challenges—to those like me who had little else to grasp onto.

I wrestled with the duality of that hope. Was I being naive? Could I truly trust an institution steeped in traditions that had not always been welcoming to Black Americans? The generational stories of disenfranchisement and discrimination were not lost on me. My father's stern warnings echoed in my mind—tales of battlefields abroad, yes, but also of internal battles waged in ranks, where color often dictated loyalty and safety. Yet, more than any lingering doubt, the desperation to escape held sway. The consequences of remaining trapped in my neighborhood were all too vivid in my mind: friends lost to violence or addiction, family members trapped in cycles of hardship, futures extinguished before they could even begin.

Emotions swirled tangled within me—fear, hope, anger, and a burning resolve that the military might finally offer the chance to claim ownership of my own destiny. For all its imperfections and dangers, it represented an alternate reality, a difficult but possible way forward. I visualized myself as more than a product of my environment, more than a statistic swallowed by the systemic failures around me. I imagined discovering my own strength, building a resilience that could withstand whatever life flung my way. The uniform symbolized possibility, honor, and a break from the insidious pattern of struggle that had defined the lives of those I loved.

In the quiet moments before making that fateful choice, the weight of my environment pressed down with relentless force. I knew the risks involved in enlisting—both those spoken and those whispered in troubled shadows—but I was equally certain of the risks in staying. The alternative was a slow death of dreams, an endless march through days cleaved thin by fear and limited chances. I could feel the invisible walls closing in around my existence, and the military stood as the only door that might swing open, revealing something bigger, something freer. Yet beneath the surface of that hope lay an unspoken truth: I harbored a fragile trust in a system that had yet to prove its capacity for fairness or protection. The idealism of youth blended with the pragmatism of survival, forming a fragile resolve to make the military the crucible in which I would forge a new self, even if it came at great cost.

The day I finally spoke the words—telling my family of my decision—was laden with an uneasy mix of pride and anxiety. Their cautious support was tinged with concern, as their love sought to armor me against the unknown dangers that lay ahead. I knew their fears were not unfounded, and yet their hope seeped through cracks in the wary facade. In their eyes, I saw reflections of their own yearning for stability and dignity, hopes they passed along to me as sacred legacies. I carried their dreams with me into recruitment centers and physical exams, every step underscored by the tension between aspiration and apprehension.

As I walked through the door of the recruitment office that first time, dressed in clothes far removed from uniforms, I felt a surge of conflicting emotions—excitement at the adventure and promise ahead, mingled with the weight of the unknown that lurked just beyond the threshold. I imagined the camaraderie of training, the pride of serving, and the possibility of learning skills that could lift me out of obscurity. Yet I also felt the silent echo of warnings—stories of those who had faced not only external enemies but internal betrayals. Still, the decision had been made; the die was cast. In that moment, all the uncertainty and anger and hope condensed into a single resolve: to grasp with both hands the chance to become something more than my past had dictated.

The military was a gamble, but it was mine, a path chosen out of an urgent need to escape entrapment and violence. It was a decision carved from pain, resilience, and the unyielding hope that somewhere amid the ranks, among strangers and trials, I would find a new beginning. Little did I know then the depths of that trial, the darkness I would face beyond the barracks, and the scars that would forever mark my journey. Yet the choice to enlist was the first step—not just away from a crushed childhood, but toward a story that would force me to confront betrayal, survival, and eventually, healing. It was the courageous, complicated decision of a boy desperate to reclaim his life and carve out a future brighter than the shadows that sought to define him.

Chapter 2
Boot Camp Beginnings

Arrival and Orientation

The bus rumbled relentlessly against the cracked pavement as it carried me further away from everything familiar—the worn streets of my neighborhood, the flickering streetlights casting uneasy shadows on graffiti-stained walls, the faint but persistent echoes of distant sirens and shouted insults. Everything I had ever known was shrinking behind me with every mile, replaced by the daunting silhouette of the military base looming ahead, a stark contrast to the familiar chaos I was trying to escape. I sat quietly, clutching the small duffle bag my mother had packed with hurried hands and whispered blessings, the tension in my stomach knotting tighter with every turn the road took. I told myself this was the beginning of a new life, a fresh start, a chance to break free from the suffocating grip of poverty, gang violence, and the crushing weight of systemic racism that had shadowed my every step. Yet, beneath those hopeful thoughts, an indistinct sense of unease settled—a whisper that maybe, just maybe, this new world wouldn't be as welcoming as I dreamed.

Stepping off the bus onto the tarmac, the air was crisp, charged with a strange mixture of sterility and discipline. The sprawling base felt both alien and oppressive, vast and meticulously ordered. Rows upon rows of identical barracks stretched into the horizon, each one a square of strict hierarchy and institutional rigor. The buzz of shouted commands, the clang of boots on hard surfaces, and the staccato rhythm of drilling soldiers filled the air like a relentless drumbeat, syncing every heartbeat into a collective cadence of conformity. The orientation center was a temporary sanctuary from this overwhelming new world—a place where young recruits like me were processed through a series of humiliations disguised as "training," brutal lessons about obedience and endurance that tore down any vestiges of individuality we carried in. I felt like a newly plucked weed in a vast, austere garden, unsure if I would be allowed to grow or simply crushed beneath the weight of expectations.

The first days at boot camp were an assault on every sense I had. Mornings began before the sun dared to rise, with shouts erupting through the barracks and soldiers shuffling in a desperate dance between icy showers and the rigid schedule of physical training. The air reeked of sweat, disinfectant, and the cloying fear that emanated from every corner. Our drill instructors, faces carved from unforgiving stone, wielded authority like a weapon, slicing through any resistance with verbal barbs and relentless pressure. Their presence was a constant reminder that this place existed to reshape us—strip away our pasts, our fears, our doubts—and forge us into something new, something stronger, or at least that's what they said. I clung to that hope, but with every barked order and punished mistake, I felt pieces of myself fray, replaced by a numb kind of obedience designed to protect against the unknown threats we were told lay ahead.

Camaraderie, or what was presented as such, formed quickly under this brutal regime. My fellow recruits—from different towns, backgrounds, and stories—became the threads that tethered me to this strange new life. We shared whispered conversations in the dark, traded glances of support amid the endless drills, and exchanged the scant moments of laughter that punctuated the exhausting days. Yet beneath the surface, the bonds were fragile, forged not from genuine connection but from shared survival. We were competitors as much as comrades, each one fighting to withstand both the external demands and internal fears. Early moments of trust were tested by the subtle pressures to conform, to mask vulnerabilities, and to adopt the hardened facades required to navigate a culture that prized strength and stoicism above all else. The tentative friendships I began to form were like fragile glass—beautiful, but always on the brink of shattering.

As the orientation unfolded, the stark realities of military life began to seep through my initial optimism. The rigid hierarchy was not just a structure for order but a tool of control, where power dynamics dictated who had safety and who became prey. The unspoken codes of conduct, the subtle but unmistakable hierarchies between soldiers of different races and ranks, started to reveal themselves like cracks in the polished surface. Whispers circulated about hazing rituals tolerated or even encouraged, and the quiet lines drawn in the sand between units and individuals felt charged with an underlying hostility. I sensed, even in those early days, the simmering tensions that lurked beneath the supposed brotherhood—tensions shaped not just by the stress of service, but inflamed by deep-seated prejudices and unspoken threats.

The training exercises themselves were relentless and grueling, pushing our bodies to exhaustion and our minds to the edge. The days blurred into a series of ritualistic motions—push-ups until my arms shook uncontrollably, timed runs that left my chest heaving, drills repeated until precision was no longer thought but instinct. It was a brutal reminder that the military demanded total commitment, not just physically, but emotionally and mentally. I was expected to shed the vulnerabilities that had kept me safe on the streets, to adopt a new identity defined by discipline, loyalty, and unfaltering courage. But inside, the wounds of my past—the losses, the fears, the desperate longing for belonging—thrummed loudly, refusing to be silenced by sweat and shouted orders.

Yet there were moments, fleeting and precious, when the uniform and structure offered shelter from the chaos I had fled. The cadence of routine brought a strange kind of comfort; the certainty of scheduled meals, the predictability of drills, and the promise of a paycheck at the end of training felt like anchors in the storm of my life. For the first time in years, I glimpsed a path toward stability. The idea of a career, of honor, and of ultimately serving something greater than myself filled me with a fragile hope. I imagined the military as a brotherhood—a sanctuary where the bonds of shared hardship could protect me from the hatred and violence that had stalked my youth. I longed to believe in that vision, even as the shadows at the edges of camp whispered warnings I dared not yet name.

The diversity of recruits within my platoon was a quiet reminder of America's contradictions. There I was, a Black kid from the ghetto, shoulder to shoulder with others whose lives differed yet intersected beneath the same uniform. Some had come from small towns with little experience beyond farming or factory work. Others bore the scars of similar violence and trauma but carried it behind closed doors. The military's promise of equality and brotherhood felt fractured, however, when racial slurs were tossed casually during downtime, and subtle exclusions marked who was included in the inner circles. There were moments when the ease of camaraderie broke sharply against the abrasive reality of racial tension. The privileged jokes, the coded language, the casual glances that lingered too long—it all signaled that beneath the imposed equality, age-old prejudices persisted, lurking beneath the surface like an unspoken enemy ready to strike.

From my earliest days in training, I noticed how race intersected with power and vulnerability. The drill instructors, predominantly white and hardened by years of institutional culture, wielded their authority with an edge that felt both disciplinary and racialized. Mistakes I made were often met with harsher criticism than those of my white peers, and the expectations carried an unspoken pressure to prove myself, not just as a soldier but as a Black man in a predominantly white institution. It was a double bind that weighed heavily on my psyche—push too hard to fit in, and risk erasing my identity; resist, and face isolation and suspicion. The military's promise of brotherhood seemed fragile, conditional, and often perilous.

At night, when the barracks fell silent, and only the hum of the base's distant machinery persisted, I lay awake grappling with a swirl of emotions. Exhaustion battled with anxiety; hope wrestled with fear. The structure that by day seemed protective now felt claustrophobic, a cage that protected me from outside violence but left me exposed to new predators. I found myself watching my back more than ever, senses sharpened by instinct and experience. Every creak, every shadow seemed loaded with potential danger. The trust I craved was scarce, and the smiles and jokes around me often hid subtle aggressions and threats.

There was an insidious undercurrent to the military culture—an aggression veiled in rituals of initiation, in the mustering of physical dominance and psychological control, where vulnerability was synonymous with weakness, and silence was demanded above all else. The reality of power dynamics within the ranks started to bleed through cracks in the façade of discipline. Stories whispered quietly among small groups hinted at hazing worse than the physical challenges we endured, stories I tried to dismiss as rumors, but which gnawed at a dormant corner of my mind. The more I observed, the more I realized that this was not just a matter of toughening us up—it was a test of loyalty to a system that often punished difference and punished those who failed to conform to its harsh, unyielding norms.

Still, in the daylight hours, I forced myself to join in the chorus of marching boots, the synchronized calls, the chants that bound us together. I clung to the naïve hope that endurance and obedience might earn me respect and protection. I tried to erase the shadows of my past from my mind, to bury the memories of violence and loss beneath layers of uniform and discipline. Each day, I told myself this was training, that this was growth, that this was preparation for a purpose greater than myself. But deep inside, a brittleness was taking root, a fragility masked by the hard exterior I was compelled to adopt.

The truth was, the military was neither sanctuary nor salvation—it was a battleground for identity, power, and survival. In that first week, amid the pounding drills and carefully orchestrated routines, I encountered the earliest stirrings of a betrayal I could not yet name. The racial divisions that haunted American society had crept into this place of supposed unity, intertwining with a culture of violence and silence that promised to consume me if I let down my guard. I came to understand that trust in this world was a fragile commodity, that hope was a risk, and that the path ahead would require more resilience than I had ever known.

Even as the days grew longer and the tasks heavier, I found refuge in small victories—the completion of a grueling run, the quiet support from a fellow recruit who shared my background, the rare moments when a drill instructor's scowl softened into a nod of acknowledgement. These sparks of humanity kept me tethered to the belief that I could withstand the storm. But they were tempered by the growing awareness that the military's promises were layered with contradictions—that beneath the surface of disability and shared brotherhood, darker forces whispered threats that would soon shatter the fragile equilibrium I fought so hard to maintain.

As orientation stretched on, each day bringing another trial of endurance and conformity, I realized that boot camp was a crucible not only for the body but for the soul. It demanded more than sweat and sacrifice—it demanded invisibility, silence, and a surrender that I wasn't certain I was willing to give. Yet I had already journeyed too far to turn back. The memories of the streets, of lost friends and broken families, pressed me forward, pushing me to believe that somewhere beyond the drills and the orders, I could find the strength to survive and maybe even thrive. Still, a quiet voice inside warned me to keep my eyes open, to guard my heart, and to prepare for the truth that lay beneath the carefully orchestrated façade of military life—an unspoken darkness that would test everything I believed about loyalty, trust, and courage.

Training Challenges

From the moment I stepped onto the tarmac that gray morning, the air already felt thick with expectation and formality, the kind that wraps around you like a suffocating cloak. Boot camp was supposed to be a crucible—a place where boys became men, where disjointed lives were melded into the disciplined, unified body of the military. I remember holding onto that hope tightly, clutching it as if it were a lifeline. After all, here was a place immune, I believed, to the chaos that had marred my youth: the gang violence that had stalked my neighborhood like a shadow too long cast, the poverty that gnawed at every meal, the systemic racism that slashed the air thicker than the humid city grime, the crack epidemic tearing families apart with incendiary speed. Boot camp was supposed to be a fresh start, a clean slate scrubbed by sweat, drill commands, and camaraderie. But looking back, I see now how naïve I was, how ill-prepared for the storm that was waiting beneath the polished boots and ironed uniforms.

The physical demands alone tested me beyond any limits I thought I had. We rose before dawn, muscles stiff from the cold floors, bodies aching from yesterday's drills. The endless mornings were a blur of running, marching, pushing, pulling; the brutal routines designed to strip weakness away like a sculptor chiseling at a block of marble. At first, my body rebelled fiercely. My legs burned on the rough tracks as they craved rest, lungs gasped for air that felt always just out of reach, and my hands were raw from gripping rifles and heavy gear. But the biggest battle wasn't against fatigue—it was against the mental toll that clung to every grueling step. Each shouted order was synchronized with the pounding in my chest, a harsh reminder that failure wasn't an option, yet fear and anxiety tangled within me like barbed wire.

The drill instructors loomed as figures of authority, merciless yet essential, their voices booming with thunder as they broke us down to build us up. They demanded perfection and submission, while their piercing gazes never betrayed a hint of softness. I quickly learned the importance of mask-wearing—the soldier's face, stoic and unreadable—because showing vulnerability was an invitation for exploitation. While I shared fleeting smiles with some of my peers during the rare moments between hellish exercises, there was an undercurrent of tension that I couldn't ignore, a subtle divide that translated into glances cast sideways, half-murmured comments, and an unspoken hierarchy beyond rank and file. The camaraderie I had envisioned—a brotherhood forged in fire—was complicated by this invisible boundary, shadowed by the different backgrounds we came from, races, all tangled up in the military's strict, unforgiving culture.

The mental landscape of boot camp was a dual battlefield. On one side lay the relentless drive to succeed, to prove that I belonged, that I wasn't just another lost kid from the city streets. On the other side loomed a constant presence of unease, like a whisper at the back of my mind, reminding me that the world outside the barracks was still waiting with its knives drawn. Sometimes the sheer absurdity of adapting to such rigid routines hit me in waves—like how we were all expected to become interchangeable parts of a machine, where feelings and personal histories had no place. It was a place where individuality was suppressed, uniformity enforced, but beneath the surface, we all carried scars, burdens invisible to the naked eye. I felt them acutely, especially in the small moments before lights out when the day's noise faded and silence stretched out like an endless desert. I thought of my mother, worn from relentless struggle, my little brother trying to survive a world that seemed scripted for failure, and the dreams I harbored of something better for all of us.

But even as I gripped hope, a creeping realization began to unfurl—this was not a sanctuary free from the social forces that had tried to crush me before. The racial dynamics within the ranks played out in subtle, sometimes cruel ways. There were jokes veiled thinly in camaraderie, the sidelining in group tasks, and the silent judgments that bore down like invisible weights. I was a Black teenager among mostly white recruits, and though we were all supposed to be equal under that uniform, the truth seeped in between sweat-soaked shirts and morning drills. It dawned on me how racial tension and division were embedded in systems that claimed unity, how hate could wear the mask of discipline and control. I noticed the way smiles could turn cold when no one else was looking, the way certain officers' eyes lingered longer than necessary, angling to assert dominance or instill fear. It was in these moments I felt the most solitary, the most exposed, even surrounded by hundreds.

Still, amidst the exhaustion and the prickling doubt, there was something magnetic about the strict order and purpose that pulsed through boot camp. The schedules, the rules, the clear articulation of goals—they gave shape to a chaotic past, a kind of grounding that felt almost sacred. For the first time, I began to glimpse a future where my actions mattered beyond survival; where strength wasn't just a necessity but a badge of honor. The unyielding discipline promised control over my own body and mind, offered a road to reclaiming dignity lost in the cracks of the streets. My early mornings pulling myself out of the sweat-damp bunks, running alongside comrades gasping for breath, shouting in unison the cadence calls—these rituals became cracks of light pushing through the fog of my past.

Yet beneath this thin thread of hope, the cold reality was already setting in. Despite the surface-level appearance of brotherhood, I sensed undercurrents of hostility that went unspoken, simmering beneath the boot camp's artificially imposed harmony. The military culture, rigorous and unforgiving, was also a powerful vessel for the very prejudices I was trying to outrun—racial bias, fear of difference, and the violent assertion of power. It was a culture that forbade questions and punished weaknesses, one where power could be wielded mercilessly behind closed doors. The early camaraderie was broken by the tension of unsaid fears and the shadows cast by those lurking within the ranks, members of hate groups infiltrating the very institution sworn to protect and serve. It was as if the structure meant to shelter us also hid predators in plain sight.

Among the chaos of commands and drills, that knowledge felt like poison seeping into my veins. Every glance that lasted too long, every smirk that slipped just beneath the surface of polite conversation, fed a gnawing dread. Boot camp was no longer just a trial of endurance—it was a minefield fraught with danger that I wasn't yet ready to face. Still, I forced myself to keep moving forward, to stay strong, to believe in a tomorrow shaped by courage rather than fear. The physical pain and mental strain blurred into one, a relentless treadmill pushing me to the edge, yet I clawed my way inch by inch, day by day, clinging to the hope that I could survive what was to come.

The weight of expectations pressed relentlessly, not just from the officers and drill instructors but from within myself. I felt the eyes of my family, the hopes of my community, and the ghosts of my past disasters all riding upon my shoulders. What they didn't see was the fragmenting fissures under the surface, how the rigid walls of boot camp were closing in, how the promise of safety and belonging was tinged with the uncanny feeling that I was stepping into a different kind of battlefield. I wanted to trust the system that would haul me out of my old life, but with every forced smile and every grueling physical test, a silent alarm echoed through the corridors of my mind, a warning of storms beneath still waters.

But I was still young, still hopeful in ways that would soon be shattered. Those weeks of training hammered into me lessons far beyond those drilled in physical endurance and military decorum—they began to teach me the harsh necessity of vigilance, the complexity of belonging in a place where brotherhood coexisted with danger. This duality became the shadow I carried into every formation, every night in the barracks, every whispered conversation under the veil of darkness. I learned, too soon, that trust in this world was both precious and perilous—a lesson paid for in silence and suffering I had yet to understand. The challenges of boot camp were not just the strain on my body or the rigors of discipline, but the awakening to an environment where hope and betrayal were intertwined, threads in a tapestry far darker than I had imagined when I first enlisted.

Building Bonds

The first weeks at boot camp arrived like a wave crashing relentlessly against the shore, battering every ounce of certainty the young man once held about his future. From the moment he was thrust into the rigid confines of military life, the day-to-day routine became an unyielding sequence of orders, drill commands, physical tests, and intense scrutiny. Yet amid the harshness and pressure, something unexpected began to take shape — the fragile tendrils of friendship that promised a kind of brotherhood, that tentative refuge amid the storm. It was in this crucible of sweat, shouted commands, and collective discomfort that bonds began to forge themselves, not out of casual choice, but necessity. The military, as much as it demanded obedience and absolute commitment, also thrived on these brotherly connections, woven tightly into the fabric of every unit. For a teenager who had grown up surrounded by chaos—gang signs, poverty, and systemic neglect—this prospect was both unfamiliar and oddly comforting.

In the early days, before the weight of the uniform settled fully on his shoulders, he clung to the hope that the military would be a place of growth and belonging. The stark contrast from his previous life could not have been more pronounced. In his neighborhood, trust was a rare currency, often overshadowed by suspicion and survival instincts. Here, in the barracks, amid strangers who suddenly became comrades, the shared struggle fostered something akin to kinship. The midnight inspections, grueling physical fitness tests, and relentless schedules that ground them down also wove them together, binding them in a collective hardship that softened the edges of loneliness. There was an invisible thread connecting the countless faces around him—young men from all walks of life, all carrying their own burdens, their own reasons for enlisting. As sweat mingled and voices rose in unison during the countless drills, a chorus of shared experience echoed louder than their individual differences.

Many of these friendships sprang up during small, stolen moments—waiting in line for chow, trudging across the training grounds, or sharing stolen smiles during moments when the drill sergeant's gaze glanced elsewhere. These fleeting interactions carried an extraordinary weight. In boot camp, where vulnerability was considered weakness, these subtle signs of mutual understanding became vital. He quickly learned to recognize the look of silent agreement, the shared smirk after a minor victory over an exhausting drill, or an arm draped casually over a hesitant shoulder in moments of doubt. The sense of brotherhood was being carefully tended in these exchanges, creating pockets of affinity that held the battleground of rigid military life at bay. Amid the shouting and discipline, he found himself confiding, quietly, to a few trusted peers—others like him, navigating the rough waters of this new existence with tentative steps.

The irony of this brotherhood was that, even in its earnest formation, it did not erase the stark realities of the deeper fractures in military culture. While the surface shimmered with camaraderie and teamwork, behind closed doors lay tensions, some simmering invisibly while others boiled openly. The young man's initial impression was shaped by hopeful yearning—he wanted to believe that the promises of equality and mutual respect would transcend the uniforms and ranks. And yet, little by little, the undercurrent of racial friction began revealing itself like cracks in an otherwise solid facade. The base was a microcosm reflecting broader society's divisions; sometimes subtle, other times blatant, the prejudices were woven tightly alongside the discipline and unity he was urged to embrace. Though this dissonance was not immediately evident to a newcomer overwhelmed by the blitz of training and adaptation, it brewed beneath every shared meal, every forced camaraderie, ready to rupture when least expected.

In those first days and weeks, the young man was painfully aware of being the "other" — the Black teenager from the city in a world where most around him were white and conditioned by histories and perspectives far removed from his own. Some in his unit made no effort to hide their disdain, their taunts cloaked as jokes, their aggressive posturing a constant reminder that acceptance was not guaranteed, that brotherhood could be fractured by something as basic as skin color. And yet, he also encountered moments of unexpected solidarity, rare but deeply vital. His closest companions were not bound just by rank or drill but by shared experiences of marginalization as much as by the grueling demands of the regime. There was a fellow recruit, smaller in frame but fierce in spirit, whose quiet defiance against the system mirrored his own. There was another, older and rugged, who softened when he spoke of his troubled past, recognizing in the young man's eyes a spark of survival he knew well. These fragile alliances helped him weather the hostile overtures from others, transforming the barren terrain of boot camp into a space where some semblance of family began to take root.

As days bled into nights, and the rhythm of boot camp became a metronome marking endurance rather than merely time, the young man began to appreciate the importance of these friendships beyond merely passing the physical challenges. The bonds forged in sweat and fatigue created a safety net, a way to hold on when the drills and discipline threatened to pull him under. In the locker rooms and quiet corners of the barracks, stories were exchanged in whispers—of home towns, of broken families, of hopes pinned on the future beyond this intense present. These stories built bridges across differences, turning strangers into brothers who could stand shoulder to shoulder against the daunting, impersonal forces of military culture. The structure that sought to make them all uniform and indistinguishable also, paradoxically, depended on these personal connections to maintain morale and identity.

But the fragility of these burgeoning relationships was a constant shadow. The drill sergeants, masters of psychological warfare, understood the importance of control not just through fear but also through creating and then exploiting fissures among recruits. Friendships could sometimes be weaponized, manipulated to sow distrust or silence dissent. The young man observed how small misunderstandings or grievances could spiral, how loyalties were tested not just by the demands of training, but by the simmering prejudices and rivalries that lurked beneath the disciplined veneer. It was a delicate dance — to trust but not so fully as to be vulnerable, to offer brotherhood without surrendering control. This often sharpened his instincts, conditioning him to weigh every friendly gesture carefully, to read between the lines of every joke or comment. The military's promise of cohesion was often marred by these complex social undercurrents, a reminder that belonging required both courage and caution.

Despite the ever-present cracks, the experience of shared hardship broke down many barriers. The endless hours spent pushing through pain during physical training blurred distinctions and forced an equality born of necessity. When muscles ached and lungs burned under the noon sun, it no longer mattered where someone came from or what prejudices they carried in their hearts — survival became the truest leveler. In training exercises, strategizing for the next drill, and helping each other through the physical tests, the young man found moments when the race or background of the other recruits melted away into a unity forged on the battlefield of endurance and sweat. This unity was both fragile and rare, a glimpse into what military brotherhood could mean beyond the surface. It planted a seed of hope that maybe in this harsh new world, he could find the stability and acceptance he sought.

Yet alongside this hope, there was an acute awareness that the bonds he was forming came with an unspoken price. Brotherhood in the military often demanded conformity—to hierarchy, to the unyielding rules, but also to the prevailing attitudes and the culture of silence. To be part of the unit was to wear its identity fully, to accept its triumphs and its hidden wounds. While friendship among recruits was a source of strength, it was also fraught with risk, especially for someone already vigilant against the racial hostility that shadowed many interactions. The need to protect oneself and one's dignity meant carefully balancing openness with guardedness. Every moment of connection was underscored by the possibility of betrayal or exclusion, a tension that lingered beneath the surface of the hardest laughs and camaraderie.

This reality was brought home in countless subtle ways. Offhand remarks during downtime, coded language that carried biting weight, a shared silence whenever certain topics surfaced — all revealed the limits of inclusion imposed by a military culture still grappling with deeply entrenched racial and social divisions. The young man learned that some wounds were invisible but no less sharp, that trust had to be earned and guarded with vigilance. Still, what kept him tethered to hope was the knowledge that the few true friendships he nurtured offered something worth fighting for—an oasis of acceptance in a world that too often had denied him such grace. In those moments, the promise of brotherhood was no longer just a vague ideal but a lived reality, a lifeline amid the imposing shadow of the military institution.

The rigorous structure of boot camp, harsh though it was, also demanded consistency and predictability, which contrasted with the chaotic unpredictability of the life he had left behind. This juxtaposition fed his initial optimism—the idea that military life, with all its strictness, could offer him a way out, a path to something better. The uniforms, routines, and clearly defined roles were grounding in a way that the fragmented, unpredictable gang-ridden streets of his youth never had been. It was the clarity and order that gave shape to his hopes for the future. With every roll call and uniform inspection, he convinced himself that this was a process not of breaking him down, but of building him up into the man he wanted to become. His friendships, too, became part of that scaffolding — together, they could navigate the complexities of military culture and survive the challenges ahead.

Yet, beneath this hopeful exterior—even as bonds deepened—there remained an undercurrent of unease. Despite the apparent brotherhood, certain recruits held stubborn biases that occasionally surfaced in hostility or exclusion. Whispers in the barracks hinted at loyalties to ideologies that clashed violently with his very existence. The distant but persistent presence of hate groups hidden within military ranks was an unspoken threat that would soon shatter whatever illusion of safety he had clung to. The very men whose friendship he sought would, in some cases, betray that fragile trust in the most brutal and devastating ways. The recognition of this lurking danger was something the young man could not fully comprehend yet, but it settled in the pit of his stomach—a shadow stretched long and dark across the horizon of his military journey.

In the final tally of those formative weeks, the bonds built in boot camp were both a lifeline and a reminder of the paradox of military life—a place where camaraderie and cruelty coexist, where strength is often born from vulnerability but can just as easily be weaponized against you. The young man emerged from this intense initiation different than when he had entered, tempered but not yet broken, carrying the weight of new friendships forged in the heat of shared struggle, alongside the bitter taste of racial divisions simmering beneath the surface. These early connections would be the foundation of his experience, shaping not only his survival but the painful journey ahead — a journey marked by betrayal, trauma, and ultimately, a search for healing beyond the bonds of brotherhood he first believed the military held.

Chapter 3
Dark Shadows Emerge

Trust Shattered

The night air was thick with a silence that seemed almost conspiratorial, the kind of quiet that presses insidiously against your skin, making every breath feel like a whispered secret you're forced to keep. I had no idea how quickly everything would unravel, how the space I thought was safe—a place where I had bet everything—would turn into the darkest trap I'd ever known. The barracks room was dim; the flickering overhead light barely pushing back the shadows pooling in the corners. I remember feeling a strange mix of emotions—a nervous hope clinging to the edges of an undercurrent of exhaustion. Hope that maybe, just maybe, here I could find a semblance of belonging, a brotherhood to lean on that I so desperately needed to grasp.

Then they showed up. Four white men, faces cold and unfeeling as stone; their movements precise, predatory. When I recognized them, those don't belong here tattoos and the subtle symbols etched onto their clothes and belongings, it froze me in a way that went beyond the physical. They were members of the Klan, the hate group that lurked like a sickness beneath the surface of our ranks, infecting the very institution sworn to protect us all.

The moment of betrayal came swift and brutal, merciless like the crack hit that once tore through my neighborhood back home. They didn't just invade my space—they collided with my trust, my body, my soul. I remember the cold metal of the door latch snapping shut behind them, sealing me in with those four ghosts of every nightmare I'd ever buried deep. Their fingers were rough and unforgiving, tearing at the lines I'd drawn to safeguard my dignity. The mop stick they wielded wasn't just a weapon; it was a declaration—a twisted symbol of both physical and psychological domination. The sickening feeling of that wooden shaft penetrating me was a violation that reverberated far beyond the pain in my body. It was a cracking of everything inside, a catastrophic rupture of the fragile faith I had placed in the uniform, the system, the people who were supposed to serve alongside me.

Their voices were cold, dripping with venom wrapped in threats so vile that they tethered me to silence. "Say a word, you're dead, and your family's next," one growled, the words slithering through the air sharper than the mop stick's impact. There was no room for negotiation, no edge of mercy in their tone—only the hard, raw calculus of hatred. I could feel my heart hammering against my rib cage, a frantic drumbeat syncing with the cold sweat slicking my skin. Fear settled over me like a suffocating cloak; not just fear for my own survival, but a terror so primal that it gnawed at my bones—the terror that the nightmare I was living was not only real but had reached inside my worst dreams to twist and distort them further.

In that dark, suffocating moment, trust shattered like brittle glass underfoot. The very foundation of what I had clung to slipped away, fracturing into countless shards that embedded themselves in my psyche. Every hope, every belief that the military could be my refuge from the violence and systemic cruelty I'd fled, was undone brutally and unapologetically. I wasn't just wounded in body; I was gouged out at the core—torn loose from the fragile thread of safety woven through rage, survival, and hope. I was left raw and exposed, swallowed by a dreadful solitude that no one could pierce unless I chose to reach out.

The immediate aftermath was a blur of shock and an intense nausea that rose like a bitter storm in my gut. My mind raced, scrambling to piece together the fragments of what had just happened, trying desperately to convince myself it was a nightmare from which I would awaken. But it wasn't. It was chillingly real, an imprint of violence branded onto my memory, forever entwined with the uniform I had once worn with pride. I slumped against the cold wall, body trembling—not from the cold, but from the sheer weight of betrayal pressing against every ounce of strength in me.

There was a terrifying silence that followed—a void filled neither by the camaraderie I expected nor by the justice I so desperately needed. Instead, an oppressive stillness settled in the room, as if the space itself had absorbed the darkness and was holding it close like a secret too dangerous to share. The unspoken message hung heavy: speak out, and the consequences would unravel beyond this moment, burning through everything I loved, everything I was still fighting to protect. It pinned me there, a prisoner of silence enforced not just by fear, but by an insidious promise that my pain would echo across the delicate threads connecting me to my family, my community, my very life itself.

In the sweeping chaos of my thoughts, I felt a heralding of betrayal that cut deeper than any physical wound: the betrayal by men sworn to uphold honor and protect, who instead exploited their power to inflict pain. They turned what should have been a sanctuary into a battleground drenched in fear and hatred. Their actions weren't just an attack on my body; they were an assault on every bond of trust that holds an army together, every unspoken vow of loyalty and brotherhood I had believed in when I raised my hand to enlist. This shattering was not isolated—it was systemic, a dark undercurrent flowing through the veins of the institution and threatening to drown anyone caught within its reach.

The psychological impact was seismic. In those early moments, confusion tangled wildly with shame and terror, creating a suffocating knot of emotions that I had no tools to untangle. I questioned everything—not just what had happened, but who I was, where I stood, and whether I had any claim left to safety or identity. The assault fractured my sense of self, splintering the once clear lines between victim and survivor, innocence and complicity, hope and despair. How do you reconcile your existence when the very place you sought solace becomes the site of your deepest violation? How do you hold onto a shattered identity when every piece screams betrayal?

As the night stretched on, I lay on the hard cot, the cold seeping into my bones, numbness slowly creeping in to dull the sting. But the numbness was a double-edged sword; it was both a refuge and a prison. It shielded me from the crushing reality but also locked me inside my own torment. Tears welled and spilled, yet they carried no relief. The weight of silence pressed down heavier with each passing hour, and I felt myself closing off from the world, retreating into an inner void where the assault replayed endlessly on loop, etched in every fiber of my being.

In those first hours after the assault, the military around me transformed from a place of discipline and order into a labyrinth of shadows and whispers. I realized with gut-crushing clarity that the threat wasn't only the men who attacked me; it was the system that allowed them to exist within its ranks, to carry out such violence with impunity. Trust, once abundant and flourishing in my heart like a fragile seedling, withered under the toxic weight of silence, fear, and institutional neglect. I felt utterly alone, isolated not only by the trauma I endured but by the walls erected by indifference and denial.

The threat to my family lingered in the corners of my mind—the ghosts of my assailants' words chaining me to a silence that felt like a slow suffocation. I thought of my mother, my little brother, the relatives back home in the neighborhood riddled with gang wars and poverty that I had fled. The thought of anything happening to them chilled me to the core, a relentless reminder of my entrapment. My body might have been violated, but so too had my sense of safety, my concept of family as an inviolable refuge. The men had invaded not only my personal sanctum but the delicate network of love and protection I'd fought so hard to maintain.

It was an unforgivable moment in time—a cruel fracture where the narrative of my life veered sharply from hope to despair. The assault was not just an event; it was a rupture that tore open every layer of trust I had built in my young life, exposing me to a loneliness and vulnerability so raw it threatened to consume me. The immediate aftermath wasn't filled with anger or justice, but with a creeping, suffocating dread that seeped deeper than any wound could go, nesting in my psyche and laying claim to my spirit. This moment marked the death of the soldier I wanted to be, and the painful birth of a survivor shackled by trauma.

The betrayal was complete—by the institution, by my peers, by the very ideals I had once held sacred. In that crucible of darkness, I was forced to confront the horrific reality that the military, a place I had joined to escape hate and violence, could also be the stage where racism, hatred, and sexual violence collided in the most devastating of ways. This was not just a personal tragedy; it was a symptom of a broken system that turned a blind eye to the pain inflicted within its walls. As the night morphed into morning, the silence was not a reprieve but a reminder that my ordeal was far from over—and that the true fight for survival had only just begun.

The Threats

The moment they cornered me, the air around us shifted with an unbearable weight, thick and suffocating, as if the night itself conspired to swallow whatever hope I clung to. The four of them— white men, insignias barely concealed but dripping with hatred— loomed over me like shadows made physical, their faces twisted by malice and a calculated cruelty that chilled my bones far deeper than the cold night air. They moved with an eerie coordination, each step echoing against the cold metal walls of the barracks, a rhythm that pulsed like a death march. I was frozen, paralyzed by disbelief and terror, my body betraying me in the most profound way even as my mind scrambled to resist, to push back, to scream. But the screams died in my throat because with them came the first words—whispers that grew into snarls—dark promises etched with violence, soaked in venom. "You don't say a damn thing," one snarled, his voice low, like a viper ready to strike. "Say a word, and it won't be you who pays."

They circled me like predators, the atmosphere electric with menace, every glance laden with the unspoken but understood threat. It was as if the very air around them conspired to mute my voice, suffocate my cries, to obliterate any flicker of defiance. The mop handle—a grotesque instrument of their cruelty—became a symbol of their power, an extension of their hate. The assault itself was a brutal, degrading act of violence, physical and psychological, forever changing the landscape of my soul. As pain seared through me, the physical agony was almost secondary to the horror of what their words implied, the cold certainty of their threats that followed like a dark cloud shadowing any chance of truth or justice. They told me plainly that my silence was non-negotiable—that speaking out meant not only the destruction of me but the annihilation of those I cared about most. Family, friends, the fragile ties that kept me tethered to who I was before this nightmare—they would all be collateral damage if I dared to breathe a word.

In the aftermath, the room seemed to shrink around me, the walls inching closer, suffocating and relentless, echoing their threats with a cruel reverberation that gnawed at my mind. That night, the world became a place not of sanctuary but of torment; the place I had sought for safety, stability, and belonging was instead the ground where my soul was ravaged and shackled by fear. The silence they enforced was an invisible chain, binding me to a prison built not of bars but of dread and shame. Their words, cold and ruthless, seeped into the cracks of my being, planting seeds of helplessness that would sprout into profound isolation. I realized then with a devastating clarity that my survival depended not just on keeping their dark secret but on navigating an endless maze of shadows where every glance, every whisper, every encounter was tinged with the threat of exposure and vengeance.

The weight of their threats was an omnipresent storm cloud shadowing every step I took; it wasn't just fear for my own well-being that gripped me—it was the gnawing terror of imagining the fallout if those threats were ever realized. I lay awake many nights afterward, replaying the incident over and over, the echo of their voices a savage chant ringing in my ears. I grappled with a rage so fierce it burned through the numbness, but was quickly smothered by the paralyzing fear of retribution. This trauma was not only carved into my flesh but tattooed onto my psyche, a permanent mark of betrayal and degradation that no amount of courage could erase easily. I became painfully aware of the twisted irony: seeking refuge had led me into the belly of a beast that sought to consume me entirely. The assault was only the beginning; the real nightmare was the captivity of silence, the forced muteness born of their threats, which strangled my voice and erased my existence.

These threats bent and distorted every thought I had, turning hope into despair, courage into cowardice. They reduced me to a husk of the person I once was—silent, fearful, and utterly alone in a crowd of indifferent faces. The military, which I had imagined as a brotherhood where loyalty and trust prevailed, revealed itself as a battleground not only of war but of hatred, racism, and an insidious system that protected predators under the guise of order and discipline. The veil of uniform and authority became a mask for barbarity, allowing those men to wield their hate with impunity, safe behind walls that prioritized their rank and skin color over the truth. Every glance at their insignias was a reminder of my powerlessness, every unspoken threat a nail in the coffin of my trust.

I wrestled with the crushing silence that bound me, feeling it grow heavier with each passing day, carving gulfs between me and my fellow soldiers who remained oblivious or willfully blind. The fear kept me distant, defensive, a shadow pressed into the corners of the room, watching, listening, always calculating ways to avoid confrontation or suspicion. I became an expert in concealment, mastering the art of invisibility in a world where my greatest danger was exposure. Even as the trauma ravaged me internally, the exterior had to remain tightly controlled, stoic—a soldier smiling for the drill sergeant, going through exercises, pretending to belong. Meanwhile, inside, a war raged on, fought in silence and solitude, the promise of death by their hands or the slow decay of my spirit a constant companion.

Their threats transcended the immediate moment of violence; they were carefully crafted tools to ensure a lifelong sentence of subjugation beyond physical pain—an unending psychological torment that followed me back to my bunk, into my dreams, into the fragile spaces where my mind tried to find solace. I felt myself withdrawing more and more, isolating from the others, refusing to let anyone see the cracks forming beneath my skin. Sometimes, I wondered if succumbing to that silence was the only way to keep the people I loved safe, to maintain some semblance of control in a world that had turned brutal and incomprehensible. But with every day that passed, that silence screamed louder, a prison of self-imposed exile etched with fear and shame so profound it colored my entire existence.

I recall vividly the suffocating nights when I would lie awake, haunted not only by what happened but by the cold certainty that these men, hidden behind authority and privilege, wielded an unspoken license to destroy anyone who dared threaten their power. Could the system that promised protection from outside threats also guard me from those within, or was I forever doomed to walk alone with this dark secret? The question gnawed at me with cruel persistence, its answer lost in a labyrinth of denial, fear, and betrayal. Even when I gathered fragmented moments of courage—tiny sparks of rebellion—I found those threats looming larger than any voice I might raise, those words a cruel echo that doused my flames before they could become a blaze.

Eventually, the psychological impact rippled beyond the boundaries of military life, invading every domain of my existence. Trust turned brittle and fragile like cracked glass; relationships with family and friends became strained under the weight of unsaid horrors and a profound inability to communicate the depths of my suffering. Addiction became a refuge—a fragile balm against the overwhelming despair—but also a trap, cementing the vicious cycle of silence and shame. Each time I numbed the pain, I also numbed the possibility of healing, increasing my isolation and desperation. The threats had corralled me into a lonely wilderness where fear ruled and hope seemed a distant, impossible dream.

Reflecting on those moments, I understand now that the threats were not random acts of intimidation but calculated weapons wielded to maintain a toxic power structure riddled with racism and violence. They were designed not just to silence me but to send a chilling message to anyone else who might dream of breaking the code of silence imposed by hate and fear. Their callous precision broke more than a body; it fractured an entire identity—my faith in humanity, the military, and myself. Yet, paradoxically, those very threats—while designed to destroy—planted seeds of resistance deep within, underground where they could not be seen but nourished a slow, painful, yet real beginning of reclaiming agency.

In the cold, dark hours after they left me there, bound by shame and fear, I realized that surviving the assault was only the first battle.

The greater fight would be against the silence, the invisible chains their threats forged, and the internalized terror that sought to stamp me into invisibility. But even in that darkest moment, buried beneath layers of dread, a fragile spark remained—a whisper of defiance that one day, somehow, I would break free from the tyranny of silence and tell my truth. This flicker ignited the slow path toward healing, a journey that demanded confronting the threats not as unbreakable shackles but as wounds that, with time and courage, could begin to mend.

The threats forced me into a stark, cruel choice—somber compliance or a perilous stand against a machine rigged to crush me— and for too long, I chose survival through silence. Yet, I came to understand that true survival would require breaking those chains, reclaiming my voice, and refusing to let the perpetrators' threats define the rest of my life. Standing on the precipice of that understanding, I found both terrible weight and fragile hope in their words. They sought to imprison me, but in their cruelty lay the impetus for a fight beyond fear—one to regain trust, dignity, and ultimately, freedom.

Conflicted Silence

The moment the reality of the assault sank into his bones, the protagonist found himself trapped within an unbearable paradox: the need to speak collided violently with the overwhelming instinct to remain silent. As the cold grip of betrayal wound through him, its fingers tightening like shackles forged from fear and shame, his thoughts became a chaotic storm with no window to clarity. In the immediate aftermath, time lost all meaning. Minutes stretched into hours, but inside him, a heavy silence compressed every shred of sound and feeling into a suffocating void. The four men—masked not just in white robes but in deep-seated hatred—had shattered more than his body; they had violated his very sense of security and belonging. Their threat was explicit and chilling: if he dared to raise his voice, retribution would reach his family, back home in the neighborhood he had so desperately fled. That warning echoed louder in his mind than any cry for help, planting roots of terror that burrowed deeper with each passing second.

The assault wasn't merely an act of physical violence; it was a calculated annihilation of identity, dignity, and hope. In the sterile confines of the barracks, where comradeship was supposed to flourish, he now faced an abyss of betrayal by those sworn to protect, not destroy. At once, the memory coursed through him in unbearable flashes—the rough texture of the mop stick, the cold, unsympathetic stares of the assailants, their menacing chants twisted by a poisonous ideology. Each detail carved itself into his psyche, a grotesque mural painted with the colors of pain and terror. But when he sought to vocalize his horror, to unburden himself of this monstrous secret, the weight of their threat crushed the words before they could even form. Fear tethered his tongue like chains forged of lead, dragging him into a cavernous silence where the screams of his soul echoed unanswered.

Inside this silence, a fierce internal battle raged, one that no one could see or intervene in. The instinct to survive crumpled under a tidal wave of helplessness and self-loathing. Small fragments of his former self—the hopeful boy who had enlisted to escape the relentless violence of his neighborhood, the young man dreaming of honor and stability—seemed to dissolve into the suffocating fog of betrayal. The racial venom driving the violence transformed the assault into a symbolic erasure, stripping away his right to existence as a Black man in a predominantly white institution. Every nerve ending, every heartbeat whispered contradictory messages: he was invisible, yet marked; powerless, yet a target; alive, but fractured. The military, which had promised sanctuary from the open-air dangers of poverty and gangs, became an inverted hellscape of torment where silence was both a prison and a lifeline.

Conflicted silence wrapped itself around him not just as an immediate defense tactic but as a complex psychological fortress. His mind scrambled to explain the inexplicable, grappling furiously with the injustice that had ravaged his body and spirit. How could he have trusted the very system that inflicted this horror? How had he misjudged the brothers-in-arms who were supposed to shield him from the darkness? These questions circled relentlessly, devouring every ounce of his self-trust and fueling a secret, shameful spiral into isolation. He imagined the consequences, envisioning the dire punishments promised by the voices of his attackers. What if reporting this meant not only physical retribution but also social ostracism by his peers, disbelief by superiors, or worse—being labeled weak or complicit? The military's rigid structure, with its culture of toughness and silence, loomed over him like a monolith, its rules acting as invisible barbwire crafted to contain pain, not release it.

As days blurred into weeks after the assault, the protagonist found himself imprisoned within the contradictions of his own silence. The choice to remain quiet became a noose tightening steadily around his neck. He wore his silence like a second skin—rough and suffocating—but fragile enough to crack under the pressure of his emotions. Every glance from another soldier, every sound in the barracks, triggered memories of the assault or the threat that followed. Nightmares invaded his sleep, fracturing any semblance of peace. Yet during daylight hours, he mastered the art of concealment, masking the scars beneath a façade of stoicism and obedience. His body betrayed no sign of the violence inflicted upon it, but inwardly, he was unraveling. The emotional numbness that blanketed his mind was both a curse and a tortured shield, blunting pain just enough to keep him functioning, but denying him the healing power of acknowledgement.

There was an unbearable loneliness that came with harboring such a secret. The absence of confiding left the protagonist with no outlet for his shattered psyche. Friendships that once offered camaraderie felt hollow, his relationships increasingly distant and superficial. He feared that disclosure would fracture them irreparably or, worse, that he would be met with disbelief and contempt from those he hoped would understand. The interplay of racial violence and sexual assault compounded this fear, isolating him further. He felt trapped in an invisible war where the enemies were not only the few who had violated him but also the countless invisible forces of systemic racism and military indifference that enabled such atrocities to occur. His silence was a testament not to consent but to survival—a desperate bid to protect what little remained of his fractured life.

The psychological aftermath twisted inside him, coiling into a dense knot of self-blame and confusion. In moments of twisted clarity, he wondered if there had been something he could have done differently, some way to prevent the nightmare. The voice of the perpetrators—white supremacists cloaked in the vestiges of military authority—echoed in his mind with venomous certainty that he was powerless and that any resistance would be futile. The betrayal inflicted was pure violence, but also a weaponized form of terror designed to silence and dehumanize him, especially as a young Black man seeking refuge in an environment that should have been structured to protect him. Despite the corrosive effects of this terror, a small flicker of resistance remained deep within—a barely perceptible ember of a desire to reclaim his story and find his voice again, even as the silence pressed down with unbearable weight.

Silence, in this crucible of trauma, was both a cage and a tentative shelter, and it shaped the contours of his suffering in ways words could not encapsulate. The silence became a living thing, an oppressive presence that infiltrated every moment, suffusing even the mundanity of daily tasks and interactions. It morphed into a shadow companion, a constant reminder of what had happened and what could still happen if he ever dared to defy the imposed muteness. His mind oscillated between the raw, vivid pain of the memories and the crushing waves of denial that sought to erase them. In these cycles, reality was fluid, unstable, and overwhelming. He felt frightened not only of the physical consequences but of the social and psychological ruptures that disclosure could unleash. The very idea of "speaking out" felt like a dangerous defiance, one that could provoke a violent backlash or shatter the fragile sense of order he tried desperately to maintain.

Yet beneath this fragility lay an unyielding desire for justice, understanding, and connection. Though silence ruled his days and nights, poisoning his relationships and eroding his self-esteem, it also nurtured a complex internal dialogue steeped in pain, anger, and confusion. He wrestled with who he was before and after that night—the boy who sought safety and the man broken in its absence. The silence forced him into solitude, but it also constructed a landscape fertile for reflection and the slow, painful germination of resilience. Despite the overwhelming odds, the conflict within him suggested that silence was not absolute; it was contested and fraught with contradictions, embodying both submission and resistance, pain and survival.

In this great struggle, the protagonist began to realize that silence was not merely the absence of sound but an active, living burden that held him captive. It was a betrayal imposed by his attackers but also a complicated response to the systemic failures around him. The military's insidious culture of silence, its failure to address racism and MST openly and effectively, compounded his isolation and suffering. This recognition seeded a nascent awareness that speaking out was not solely about personal healing; it was a radical act of defiance against an institution that had, in many ways, turned its back on him. Yet the choice to break the silence was agonizing, shadowed by the still-looming threats and his own doubts. His voice was fragile, trembling with the weight of truth and fear, a voice caught between the desire to expose and the instinct to hide, reluctant but growing in strength.

Thus, the conflicted silence was not one-dimensional but saturated with layers of meaning and feeling. It was born of trauma, shaped by racial hatred, fueled by terror, and sustained by a complex psychological interplay of denial, shame, fear, and hope. He understood that lifting the veil on this silence would be an act of bravery beyond mere words—it would mean confronting not only his assailants but the entrenched systems and attitudes that allowed such violence to fester unchecked. And yet, even as he clung to silence out of necessity and dread, a quiet voice beneath the noise whispered that healing, though distant, was still possible. The decision to keep silent was not final, but a painful step on an arduous path marked by uncertainty, resilience, and the flickering possibility of reclaiming his voice and his life from the ruins of betrayal.

Chapter 4
Living with the Secret

Emotional Turmoil

The days that followed the assault unfolded as if the world around him had been irreversibly shattered into jagged fragments, each edge sharp with a pain that no balm could soothe. The immediate shock of the trauma gave way to a churn of emotions so overwhelming and contradictory that he found himself lost in their ceaseless swirl. At first, numbness engulfed him like a merciless fog, a desperate defense mechanism his mind conjured to shield itself from the raw, undeniable truth of what had happened. His body was alive with pain, bruises, and scars that would fade with time, but it was the invisible wounds lodged deep within his psyche that clawed at his soul relentlessly. Night after night, the memories replayed in an unending loop behind his closed eyelids, the horrific image of those four men—their faces twisted with cruel satisfaction—etched indelibly in his mind. Their threat against his family hung like a noose around his neck, suffocating hope, binding his voice in chains of terror and silence.

The psychological landscape into which he had been plunged was hostile, desolate, and disorienting. Trust, once an implicit thread in every relationship he held or would attempt to form, frayed into dust. The comradeship and brotherhood he had longed for as an escape from the suffocating violence and rejection of his neighborhood now felt like a distant mirage, forever beyond his grasp. Paranoia seeped into his consciousness, turning even the simplest interactions into minefields. Every glance, every whispered comment felt like a veiled threat or a judgment waiting to be cast. His world contracted into a solitary cell constructed by fear and shame, where isolation was both a prison and a refuge. Friends who had once seemed solid pillars quietly drifted away, not out of malice but the incomprehension that often greets pain too profound to bear. He could not articulate the complicated cocktail of betrayal and humiliation he carried, and in that silence, the gulf between himself and others widened irreparably.

Unable to find solace in the camaraderie he had hoped for and too terrified to disclose the trauma for fear of retaliation, he turned inward, clutching at the few fragments of control he could still command. The once-confident teenager who had believed in the military as a path to a better life became a shadow, haunted and hollow. He began to navigate his days with a shell over his heart, an emotional armor forged from distrust and dread. Inside, however, turmoil brewed with unrelenting ferocity. Flashbacks would strike without warning, plunging him back into the nightmare, triggering waves of nausea and panic. Sleep became elusive; when it came, it bore no respite. Nightmares were frequent visitors, blurring the boundaries between past horror and fragile present. The agonizing tension of waiting for an inevitable betrayal, the gnawing fear for his family's safety, and the deep wound of violated dignity coalesced into a storm too violent to weather alone.

In an effort to quell this tempest, he sought out the sedatives of various vices, gravitating first toward alcohol, then descending into drugs that promised an escape from the relentless ache inside. These substances, alluring in their promise of numbness and oblivion, initially provided brief interludes where the noise of torment would dull or retreat. Yet, as the days slipped by, the temporary relief morphed into dependency. The lines between using to forget and being controlled by the need blurred until addiction itself became another oppressor in his life. Each high was followed by deeper lows—despair that embraced him in its cold, unyielding grip with renewed cruelty. His body weakened, relationships crumbled, and his ambition evaporated into the ether of self-destruction.

Beneath the surface of this downward spiral beat a heart still yearning for connection, for kindness, for justice that never came. The betrayal at the hands of supposed protectors and brothers was not just a physical violation; it was a mutilation of his very sense of self and worth. The racial hatred embedded in the crime added layers of complexity to his trauma, inflicting wounds that pulsed with the centuries-old pain of systemic oppression. The knowledge that his attackers belonged to a white supremacist group within the military ranks compounded his feeling of alienation; it was as if the very institution he had entrusted to safeguard his future was a battleground for racial hatred and violence. This corrosive awareness seeped into his identity, fueling deep-seated rage and sorrow that often surfaced in moments of quiet despair. He questioned not only the loyalty of his assailants but the values and promises of an institution that had failed him so profoundly.

As time passed, the emotional cacophony—the grief, the rage, the shame, the confusion—began to erode any remaining semblance of the hopeful person he once was. Each day felt like walking through a landscape strewn with emotional landmines. Attempting to form new relationships seemed impossible when the self he encountered in the mirror was fractured and unfamiliar. He felt alien even to himself, a stranger in his own skin. The internal battle to reconcile the image of the soldier he aspired to be with the broken survivor he had become raged silently and invisibly. This dissonance drove him into isolation, deepening his sense of invisibility and abandonment.

The coping mechanisms he developed were, at best, flawed lifelines. He built emotional walls so high and impermeable that even when moments of vulnerability arose, they were crushed beneath the weight of shame and self-preservation. Crying, once a natural human outlet, was suppressed into an unbearable weakness. He learned to silence his own pain as fiercely as the threats had forced him to silence his truth. The loneliness became a cloak, shielding him from the piercing eyes of judgment and the casual cruelty of ignorance. He learned to perform normalcy, going through motions without hope or engagement. This masquerade wore thin with each passing day, revealing the rawness underneath but also protecting him from further harm.

At times, fleeting bursts of anger threatened to break loose, manifesting as outbursts that startled those around him, further severing the fragile human connections he tried so desperately to preserve. The rage was not only at his aggressors but at the system that allowed such injustice to fester, at the world that seemed indifferent, and at himself for being powerless to stop it. These emotions, untamed and misunderstood, left him exhausted and more deeply alienated. In the quiet moments when anger subsided, it was replaced by a profound sadness that threatened to drown him in despair. The duality of anger and sorrow waged war inside him, leaving little space for hope.

Compounding these internal battles was the overwhelming sense of betrayal—not just from the men who had attacked him but from the military structure that had failed to protect him and the silence that ensued. The lack of immediate support, the whispers of disbelief, and the fear of retaliation fostered an environment where victims like him were left voiceless and invisible. This institutional betrayal deepened his wounds, fostering cynicism and mistrust not only toward the military but toward authority and societal structures at large. The betrayal stretched beyond personal violation into a systemic failure that silenced survivors and perpetuated cycles of abuse. This realization settled like a heavy fog over his mind, obscuring any light that might have shone through the cracks.

His mental state during this period was fragile and volatile, a precarious balance held together by sheer willpower. He vacillated between moments of despair and brief glimpses of self-loathing masked as resilience. The pain of betrayal was not confined to the assault itself but extended into every fracture of his identity—as a Black man, as a soldier, and as a human being deserving of dignity and safety. These intersecting layers of trauma complicated his healing, making the path forward seem insurmountable. Every attempt to articulate his experience was met with the crushing weight of suspicion, victim-blaming, or silence, reinforcing his isolation and deepening the scars etched within.

Despite the engulfing darkness, beneath the layers of trauma and mistrust, there remained a faint ember of resilience—a stubborn refusal to be defined solely by victimhood. Deep within, he wrestled with the desire to reclaim agency over his life, to break free from the chains of shame and silence. But this emerging hope was fragile, easily smothered by the relentless tide of memories and fears. The complexity of his psychological landscape defied easy categorization or simplistic solutions. He was caught in the tension between survival instincts urging concealment and an innate yearning for truth and healing.

His coping mechanisms, although largely destructive, were part of a broader, unconscious struggle to assert control in a world where power had been violently stripped from him. Substance use, withdrawal, and emotional numbing were desperate attempts to reclaim agency, if only temporarily. These patterns highlighted the deep need for recognition, compassion, and effective intervention that could guide him toward a different relationship with his pain. But validation felt elusive in a system often marked by skepticism and neglect.

This internal exile was exacerbated by the racialized nature of his assault, shaping his self-perception and his distrust in ways unique and profound. The knowledge that his attackers operated within white supremacist frameworks inflicted psychological harm that intertwined personal violation with historical legacies of racial terror. The internalized impact of this racialized betrayal seeped into his everyday existence, influencing how he related to authority, community, and even his own body. Healing required not only confronting personal trauma but grappling with systemic injustices that had facilitated his victimization and obstructed justice.

In countless moments of solitude, when external distractions faded, he was left to face the vastness of his trauma. The silence was deafening, filled with the echoes of broken promises and stolen innocence. Yet, even in the midst of despair, the faint pulse of human endurance persisted. His journey through emotional turmoil was marked by profound suffering but also by the gradual awakening of a will to survive, to seek help, and to begin the slow, arduous process of reclaiming his narrative from the shadows of betrayal. The complexity of his emotional landscape was a stark reminder that trauma's scars run deep, but so too does the potential for resilience and transformation when given the space, support, and courage to heal.

Isolation and Withdrawal

Isolation crept into his life with the quiet persistence of a relentless shadow, swallowing the spaces once filled with laughter, camaraderie, and the tentative hope he'd clung to before arriving at the military base. It was as though the trauma seeping from within his fractured soul had carved a cavern around him, dark and claustrophobic, into which he gradually retreated. Each day, the distance between himself and those around him grew—not just physically, but in the vast chasm of understanding, trust, and belonging. The faces of his comrades blurred, their voices muffled echoes against the pounding drum of his internal torment. He found himself shrinking into himself, refusing the warmth of human contact because it threatened to ignite the flames of vulnerability he was desperate to snuff out. It was easier to pull away than to confront the gnawing fear that everyone's eyes concealed judgment, secrets, or worse—hostility.

Within the confines of his barracks room, he became a ghost haunting his own existence. The world beyond his door was an overwhelming tempest of noise, expectations, and unspoken rules, yet inside, silence stretched endlessly, void of comfort. His thoughts turned in circles like a caged animal desperate to escape the memories seared into his mind. The image of those four men—their faces twisted in cruel satisfaction, the harsh grip of their hands, the horror of the mop stick—replayed relentlessly, a sickening film reel he could neither fast-forward nor rewind to a gentler scene. The threat they made, a vow of harm to his family if he ever spoke, tightened around his throat like a noose, choking any cry for help before it could be heard. To reach out meant risking more than his own pain; it meant endangering those he loved. This unbearable secret turned him inward, building walls of silence so tall and thick that even his closest allies seemed like strangers drifting on the other side.

His retreat was marked by the slow disintegration of bonds forged in the crucible of shared hardship; the unspoken language of glances, inside jokes, and mutual respect with his fellow soldiers faded into absent nods and awkward silences. Conversations that once flowed freely now stumbled over barriers of suspicion and hopelessness. Where once he might have laughed or confided in a trusted comrade, now he sat in quiet corners, head bowed, eyes vacant, as if the very act of speaking would unravel him completely. Invitations were met with excuses, encouragement with indifference, and any attempt at connection was deflected by practiced nonchalance. In his mind, he weighed the risk of exposure against the desperate need for companionship; the scales always tipped towards self-preservation through solitude.

Loved ones on the outside were no refuge either. Phone calls became brief, strained affairs where he masked his turmoil behind a veneer of normalcy. The voice on the other end could not see the howling storm within, nor could he articulate what words might break the fragile illusion. The longing to share his grief clashed violently with the instinct to protect them, creating a suffocating silence that widened the gulf between them. Letters went unanswered or were avoided altogether, the pain and shame too raw to unpack for even the people who cared most. It was paradoxical—a profound yearning for connection battled with the fear that any disclosure would only burden those he loved and deepen his isolation further.

As the days blurred into weeks and months, his psyche began to adopt coping mechanisms that were both desperate and destructive. The numbness that settled over his thoughts became a merciful anesthetic against the excruciating memories. He reached for whatever substances promised escape, trailing a faint but dangerous path into the shadows of addiction. Each sip of alcohol, every hit of illicit drugs, momentarily muted the relentless whispers of trauma. They became an unspoken pact—a silent ally promising freedom through oblivion, even if just for fleeting moments. Yet, this solace came at a terrible price, clouding judgment and alienating him further from those who might have offered sanctuary had he the strength to accept it.

In isolation, the sense of alienation grew with a merciless intensity, fed by the intersection of his pain and the harsh realities of racial prejudice embedded within the very institution he had once hoped would provide sanctuary. The knowledge that his assailants were not just fellow soldiers but members of a hateful organization that thrived on white supremacy eviscerated his trust not only in people but in the system itself. The military, which had promised order and honor, revealed itself as a breeding ground for the very abuses he feared would escape. This revelation layered his isolation with bitterness, a toxic element that corroded any remnants of faith he had left. To be a Black man in an environment where the enemy was sometimes not just external but within, where systemic racism intertwined with sexual violence, birthed a profound loneliness that words could scarcely capture.

He wrestled silently with the dual wounds of betrayal by his comrades and the self-imposed exile needed to survive in the aftermath. Nights grew longer, filled with restless torment as memories collided with nightmares that blurred the line between sleep and wakefulness. Daylight brought no reprieve; the sunlight was a stark reminder of the world continuing to move on while he stood frozen in time, stuck in the haunted limbo of his trauma. His body bore invisible scars—signs of a battle fought within the confines of his own mind, a war unknown to those around him. Each gesture, each avoidance of interaction, was a shield wielded against further harm, yet it isolated him into a cage of his own making.

Within this crucible of loneliness, he found himself fragmented, a mosaic shattered by violence and fear. His identity flickered uncertainly between the hopeful youth who had once believed in a better future and the broken survivor battling despair. Emotions once vibrant—hope, trust, joy—became distant memories, buried beneath layers of numbness and shame. Yet, even at his darkest moments, there lingered a fragile thread of resilience, a quiet refusal to be consumed entirely by the shadows. This inner spark was a shadowy pulse beneath his withdrawal, an ember waiting for the breath of healing to kindle it once again.

Amid this desolate landscape, he noticed how his withdrawal created a feedback loop—alienation bred despair, and despair reinforced isolation. The more he pushed people away, the more he felt the weight of loneliness crushing his spirit; the heavier the burden, the tighter his grasp on solitude became. It was a prison constructed by fear and pain, yet maintained by an instinct for survival. This cycle was relentless, a torment from which there seemed no escape, until the slow and uncertain path to recovery began to emerge on the distant horizon.

The act of isolation, while instinctual and protective in the immediate aftermath of trauma, evolved into a complex psychological defense that exacted a heavy toll on his mental health. Depression swelled, manifesting in feelings of worthlessness and invisibility, as though he had been erased completely from the tapestry of life around him. Anxiety pervaded every interaction, transforming mundane encounters into minefields of potential rejection or harm. The once clear lines between friends and foes blurred, suspicion grew, and trust became an elusive luxury that he could no longer afford. This internal dissonance alienated him from the vibrancy of the military community and from his own sense of self, leaving a hollow shell where identity once blossomed.

He observed the world through a veil of detachment, a necessary armor that protected his fragile psyche from further injury. The laughter and solidarity of other soldiers became distant echoes, foreign and unreachable. Moments of kindness, hints of camaraderie, felt like illusions—betrayals of a trust he was no longer willing to extend. The isolation deepened not only because of fear and pain but because of a profound misunderstanding: he believed that no one could grasp the magnitude or the particular intersection of racial hatred and sexual violence he endured. This sense of otherness solidified the barriers that separated him, forging an invisible fortress around his wounded heart.

Yet, not all isolation was complete. In brief, fleeting moments, the walls he built cracked. Sometimes, in the quiet solitude of the night, when exhaustion softened the edges of his pain, he allowed himself to imagine a life beyond this prison—a life where his voice could be heard without danger, where his story would not lead to shame but to compassion. These moments were fragile and quickly suppressed, offering both hope and despair in equal measure. They underscored the complexity of human resilience—the way hope and trauma can coexist, battling within the same soul.

As he navigated this maze of isolation, he began to notice small signs of life stirring beneath the surface of his withdrawal. Occasional acts of self-care, however imperfect or sporadic, hinted at an inherent will to survive. Whether it was a momentary decision to attend a meal, a fleeting engagement with a fellow soldier's question, or a silent prayer whispered in the dead of night, these acts formed the seeds of reconnection. They were faint, often overshadowed by the enormity of his pain, but they carried the promise of emergence from the shadows.

The process of withdrawal also entailed layers of self-protection, where he learned to mask his vulnerabilities behind a stoic facade. This armor, while crucial in the hostile environment he inhabited, became a double-edged sword. It shielded him from exposure but also from genuine human connection. His laughter was hollow, his silence impenetrable, and his gaze evasive. The emotional numbness was both a curse and a refuge, a place where pain was kept at bay but where life's richness was also dulled.

Isolation, in this context, was not merely a physical state but a profound psychological and emotional separation. It was the erosion of the fundamental human need for connection and understanding. The military, with all its structure and discipline, ironically fostered a culture of silence and invisibility around such wounds. The systemic failures to acknowledge and address MST compounded the protagonist's experience of alienation, making his isolation not just personal but institutional. Every unreported incident, every dismissed complaint, every cultural blind spot deepened the fissures that separated him from possible allies and supporters.

Within this solitude, the protagonist grappled with the weight of unspoken trauma, buried deep beneath layers of fear, shame, and urgency to survive. The silence wasn't peaceful; it was stifling, an oppressive force that pushed him further into the margins of both his military unit and his own life. It was as if he had become a specter, present physically but absent emotionally, a man lost in a crowd yet utterly alone. The dissonance between his external world and internal reality widened, feeding the misconception that no one could truly understand the monstrous breach of trust he endured.

Yet, through this labyrinth of isolation and withdrawal, the faint glow of hope flickered. Unbeknownst to him at the time, this phase was a painful but necessary part of his journey—a raw and honest reckoning with trauma's hold. It was within this crucible of loneliness that the seeds of eventual healing would take root. As much as isolation represented a retreat, it also shielded him until he could find a way to reach out safely. The long, arduous process of reclaiming voice, trust, and self had not yet begun, but it would, fueled by the slivers of resilience that persisted beneath his silence.

In those dark, lonely hours, he learned an unspoken truth about survival—that sometimes the only way to endure the unimaginable is to withdraw, to become a fortress, to hide from the world in order to protect what remains inside. And though isolation threatened to consume him, it also preserved a fragile core of strength, waiting patiently for the courageous step that would shatter the silence and set him on the path toward healing and reclamation of his life.

Masking the Pain

The days following the assault blurred into nights that felt heavier than any he had ever known. At first, he tried to hold everything inside, to carry the weight of the violence and the betrayal silently, as if the sheer act of naming it might cause the walls of his world to crumble. The shame was a suffocating presence, wrapping around his chest like an iron coil. He told himself to stay strong, to survive by ignoring the storm that raged beneath the surface. But the truth was, every waking moment was punctuated by an ache that wasn't just physical—it was an erosion of his very soul. He found himself retreating into shadows, avoiding conversations and gatherings, afraid that even a glance from a fellow soldier might reveal the fractured pieces of his being. The camaraderie he once envisioned as a balm to his troubled past now felt like a distant mirage, a cruel reminder of what had been stolen. With each passing day, the isolation grew, and with it, the cracks in his resolve deepened, until he barely recognized the face staring back at him from the mirror.

In this void, substances crept in—not because he sought a solution, but because his mind desperately grasped for a reprieve from the unending turmoil. His first foray into alcohol was almost accidental, a casual drink shared in the barracks to blend in among the others, to feel momentarily unburdened from the suffocating silence that clung to him. The warmth of the whiskey burned a small path through the darkness, a fleeting distraction that dulled the edges of his pain. But that brief respite was addictive in its elusiveness, enticing him to reach deeper into the bottle night after night. It wasn't long before he found himself sneaking away during breaks to steal cigarettes, scraping together pennies to buy whatever drink he could afford from off-base stores, sometimes even hitting the local strip mall with other soldiers as a way to erase the memories that clung to him like shadows. These habits took root in his life, subtle at first, masking the torment that words could neither express nor admit. The rituals of drinking and smoking became armor, though it was fragile and flawed, a feeble attempt to shield him from himself.

But it wasn't just the alcohol; soon, marijuana entered the picture—a friendlier, more forgiving companion that seemed to offer a softer veil over the pain. The dense smoke swirled around him in the quiet hours, taming the intrusive thoughts that spiraled in his mind. It helped him retreat further into his own world, a sanctuary where the horrors of the assault felt dimmer, less immediate, less defining. Yet, as the numbness of the smoke seeped through his veins, it also deepened his alienation from the world around him. The camaraderie he once sought was replaced by solitary sessions in dimly lit corners, places where no one asked questions and no one saw the cracks beneath the surface. The substance use became a language unto itself, a secret dialogue with pain that the protagonist did not yet have the words to articulate outright. It was a slow, insidious process; he wasn't chasing intoxication for pleasure but fleeing from a reality that had become unbearable.

The weight of the trauma was relentless, and the substances only ever promised temporary reprieve. He learned to mask the pain until it was no longer about feeling better but about simply feeling anything at all. The military's structured routine, once a source of purpose, became a backdrop to his numbing rituals. Training drills, physical exercises, and assignments passed by in a haze, the hum of commands and marching steps fading into the background noise of his internal battle. Each day felt like a tightrope walk—juggling the need to fulfill his duties and the craving for the hollow comfort of intoxication. He was aware, on some level, that the more he sank into this cycle, the further he removed himself from the light of hope he once clung to. Yet, confronting the trauma head-on seemed impossible; the fear of speaking out, of exposing the horror, coupled with the threat hanging over his family, held him captive in silence. Instead, the substances became a distorted lifeline, the only tool he felt he had to stave off complete collapse.

His relationships within the military community further fractured under the weight of his growing alienation. Some comrades, smelling the change in his demeanor, offered shallow sympathies, while others recoiled or whispered behind his back, unaware of the true reasons behind his withdrawal. The biting realities of racism and hate that he'd already endured outside seemed to infiltrate the very ranks that promised refuge. Rumors and suspicions often danced in the corners of his unit's common spaces, isolating him further as he feared any misstep might expose vulnerabilities he desperately wished to hide. The men responsible for his violation remained a specter haunting every exchange, their presence a continual threat that made trust impossible. This undercurrent of violence and hatred was not always visible but shaped every interaction and shadowed every sense of intimacy. These fractures compounded the loneliness that nudged him deeper into his coping mechanisms, a spiral that felt impossible to interrupt or escape.

Beyond the walls of the barracks, his family life suffered as well. Calls home grew infrequent and strained, the cheerful voice he once offered to his mother becoming brittle and infrequent. The burden of silence was a constant weight, a secret wrapped tightly to protect those he loved from the devastation that colored every corner of his existence. The more he withdrew, the more mysterious and distant he seemed to those who could have provided comfort. His siblings noticed the shift, the way his eyes no longer held the spark of youthful hope, replaced instead by a haunted glaze. The neighborhood's familiar faces became a reminder of the past he sought to outrun, but even that refuge felt compromised now that the army, supposed sanctuary, had betrayed him so profoundly. This compounded his sense of dislocation, caught between worlds yet belonging fully to neither. The dissociation he felt was not just emotional but existential—a painful awareness that he was losing himself in the depths of trauma and substance dependence.

The nights were the hardest. Darkness brought a flood of memories and fears that the daylight hours could not fully suppress. Lying awake, he relived the assault—the crude brutality, the hateful snarls, the malice in those four faces etched forever in his mind. Despite the alcohol and drugs, flashes of that nightmare would erupt without warning, dragging him back regardless of how far he tried to run. He wrestled with invisible chains of shame and rage, helpless against the tidal waves of grief and pain. His dreams offered no sanctuary, twisted by fear and torment, blurring the line between sleep and the waking terror he fought to conceal. It was during these hours that the full weight of his alienation was felt most acutely. He was trapped in a body that had become both battleground and prison, tortured by memories that he could neither erase nor escape.

Inside himself, he was fighting a war more relentless than any drill or combat practice. The battleground was his own mind and spirit, and slowly, the defenses he had built were eroding in the corrosive acid of despair. The substances, initially masks, now felt like chains, anchoring him to a fracturing existence. Yet even in this engulfing darkness, there were flickers of resistance—brief moments when the desire to heal and reclaim his life whispered faintly beneath the chaos. However dim and fragile, these sparks hinted at a distant future where the pain might not control him anymore. They were the first shards of hope, buried deep beneath layers of torment, waiting for the day when he might finally find the strength to face the past and begin the long journey toward recovery.

As the cycle of masking and numbing continued, the protagonist's internal landscape became a tangled web of conflicting emotions. Anger simmered beneath a veneer of resignation; despair locked arms with fleeting moments of longing for normalcy. Each sip of alcohol and each drag of smoke was a plea for relief that was never permanent, a silent battle between the urge to disappear and the stubborn will to survive. The substances dulled the pain but never erased the scars. Instead, they etched new wounds in the form of dependency and deepening isolation. He became a ghost of the person he once was, moving through his days in a haze, caught between the burning need to hide and the aching desire to connect. With every step deeper into addiction, the barriers around his trauma thickened, obscuring the path to healing.

Yet, despite the growing darkness, the seeds of reclaiming his identity were sprouting somewhere beneath the rubble. Through fragmented memories of happier times and faint echoes of the dreams he once held, a small but persistent voice refused to be completely drowned out by the clamor of pain and fear. It was this voice—the essence of his humanity—that ultimately proved resilient, even as substances threatened to swallow him whole. The beginning of substance use as a coping mechanism was not a surrender but a symptom of a broken system that failed to protect him, a reflection of a young man's desperate search for peace in a world turned hostile and unfathomably cruel. This painful chapter of masking the pain was the crucible in which his story of survival and eventual healing would be forged.

Chapter ❖
Downward Spiral

Addiction Takes Hold

The days blurred into a relentless haze, a swirling fog that swallowed time and reason alike as addiction tightened its grip around his fragile spirit. What began as a fractured defense against the hollow ache inside soon transformed into an all-consuming force steering the course of his existence. The first encounter with the needle, the bottle, or the pipe was not born of whimsy or reckless indulgence but emerged from the raw, unfiltered agony left by betrayal—a wound jagged and pulsing beneath the veneer of a soldier forged in discipline and resilience. Each stolen moment of intoxication unraveled the fragile threads holding his fractured self together, inviting the spectral ghosts of that horrific night back to haunt every breath, every whispered memory, every tremor traced beneath his skin.

In the shadows of past violence, addiction found fertile ground, its tendrils extending deep into the crevices formed by pain and isolation. The bright ideals he once held—hope for a new life, the promise of camaraderie, a chance to rise above the cycles of poverty and violence—faded beneath the weight of trauma unaddressed and yearning unmet. The assaults, branded not only in flesh but carved mercilessly into his psyche, twisted his sense of safety from the military's embrace into a spiraling cage of fear and shame. Surviving became synonymous with numbing—to mute the flood of intrusive memories, to silence the ceaseless whispers of dread, to dull the sting of the past's brutal betrayal. Drugs offered that numbing reprieve, a fleeting illusion of peace and control when the world seemed otherwise unrelenting and hostile.

What began as occasional relief soon became a necessity, an insatiable craving that dictated his hours and thoughts with merciless urgency. The substances themselves mattered less than the escape they provided: whether it was the sharp slicing rush of cocaine, the heavy oblivion of heroin, or the liquor that burned through his throat like fire—each was a siren's call demanding allegiance. Dependence grew incrementally, insidiously poisoning every aspect of his life. Friends drifted away like autumn leaves scattered by a harsh wind, unable or unwilling to confront the chaos consuming him. Family ties, once resilient under the strain of hardship, began to fray under the relentless strain of broken promises, missed calls, and absences explained away by shame or denial. Housing turned unstable, relationships fractured, and hopes for a future dissolved into the urgent present marked by the next fix or the next blackout.

His mornings, if they could be called that, were often greeted with dry heaving and shaking hands, a desperate attempt to quell the tremors unleashed by withdrawal. Memories surfaced with brutal clarity during these moments—the laughter of those who violated his trust, the threat-laden eyes, the sickening inevitability of silence demanded by fear. The juxtaposition between his physical torment and his internal screams forged a chasm impossible to bridge. Yet, paradoxically, every nightfall brought with it the promise of oblivion, a descent into a false Eden shaped by smoke, pills, and drink—the only refuge from a mind ravaged by unrelenting trauma.

Addiction also warped his perception of self, gradually eroding the tenuous threads of identity that survived the assault. The boy who once ran from gang violence, the young man who bravely joined the ranks to forge a better path, seemed to dissolve beneath layers of guilt and self-loathing cultivated by abuse and compounded by chemical dependency. Each high was a fleeting victory against the darkness, but the comedown was an abyss where hope was swallowed whole. Loneliness, already a weight from his secrets and fear, grew heavier, solidifying around him like concrete. His trust in others—already shattered by racialized sexual violence and military betrayal—became a distant memory, replaced by paranoia and defensive walls built from pain and survival instincts.

The societal silence around Military Sexual Trauma only deepened his isolation. In a culture that valorized strength and stoicism, admitting weakness or victimhood was not merely discouraged; it was often met with suspicion and contempt. The racial dimensions, where African American men faced both the stigma of sexual victimization and the pervasive legacy of systemic racism, added layers of invisibility to his suffering. Within the military's rigid hierarchy, where loyalty was demanded and whistleblowers punished, he navigated a precarious existence, balancing self-preservation with the crushing weight of secrecy. Outside its gates, the chaotic world he sought to escape had not faded; rather, it mirrored the chaos inside, with drugs and despair welcoming him back into their unforgiving fold.

Homelessness followed as an almost inevitable consequence, a cruel testament to the broken safety nets meant to catch those struggling with trauma and addiction. Nights were spent huddled beneath the indifferent glow of streetlights, wrapped in tattered blankets that did little to shield him from the biting cold or the ceaseless ache of abandonment. Meals, when available, were scavenged from dusty convenience stores or from strangers whose kindness was as fleeting as the days themselves. The streets became a battleground of survival, marked by the constant threat of violence, exploitation, and further degradation—a grim echo of the violation he had endured within the military but magnified by poverty and neglect.

Addiction's demands drove him into dangerous circles, where dealers preyed on vulnerability, and false promises of relief masked the deepening abyss. The numbing haze that once provided sanctuary morphed into a tyrant's yoke, dictating his every action and reaction.

Financial desperation led to the erosion of ethical boundaries, and desperation pushed him toward desperate choices. Encounters with law enforcement, arrests, detox stints, and rehabs punctuated this bleak narrative, offering temporary respite but rarely breaking the cycle. Each relapse intensified his self-hatred, feeding an internal narrative that he was broken beyond repair—an echo of the hateful words whispered by his assailants and the military system's silent complicity.

Yet, beneath the anguished surface, faint flickers of resilience endured. Despite the maze of despair, there were moments, often fragile and fleeting, where a sliver of his former self emerged— memories of a young man hopeful for escape, dreams of a life reclaimed from darkness, and the quiet yearning for dignity and justice. Addiction may have held him in its grip, but it never entirely extinguished the possibility of healing. Somewhere within the depths of his weary heart, the seeds of recovery lay dormant, waiting to be nurtured by compassion, understanding, and the courage to confront a past too painful to face alone.

The path was neither linear nor merciful. It was marked by setbacks, deterioration, and nights where giving up seemed the easier option, where he felt invisible to the societies that surrounded him— those who failed to recognize the scars borne by survivors like him. In this abyss, the internal battle raged unceasingly: a struggle between surrender and the faint but persistent call toward survival. Addiction became both enemy and a misunderstood companion, symbolizing the broader societal failures to adequately support those shattered by sexual violence, especially when intersected by the brutal realities of race and militarism.

Life under addiction's shadow was a tumultuous sea of conflicting emotions—shame and defiance, despair and flickers of faith, weariness and stubborn tenacity. The substances, while offering momentary escape, underscored the profound void left by trauma unacknowledged. It was a void no amount of chemicals could fill, and each attempt to drown the pain deeper only sharpened the thorns embedded in his soul. Though he wandered through these dark corridors of addiction, the essence of his identity—shaped by early dreams, love, and the deep wounds of betrayal—remained buried, aching to emerge.

Thus, addiction took hold not merely as a series of poor choices or moral failings, but as a complex and painful testament to the profound impact of unchecked trauma on a young man whose life had been irrevocably altered. It was a cruel mirror reflecting the systemic neglect and silence around Military Sexual Trauma and racial violence within the military, a wider societal indictment that echoed far beyond his personal struggle. Understanding this dependency meant seeing beyond the substance use to the profound human story beneath—a narrative of survival, loss, and the arduous journey toward reclaiming a shattered self.

Losing Ground

The cold crept unnoticed at first, a subtle whisper against the thin mattress crumpled beneath me, but as the night deepened, it wrapped itself around my bones like an unrelenting vice. The pavement beneath the overpass was unforgiving, hard and ragged, building an unforgiving goblin of discomfort that toyed with sleep and sanity alike. I could hear the city breathing around me, a symphony of distant sirens, clattering garbage cans, and muffled conversations from passing cars. It was a lullaby of isolation, an eerie comfort in its familiarity. Every inch of space I claimed that night was contested—whether by the chill in the air, the ache in my joints, or the gnawing hunger that had taken up residence inside my gut. This was not the life I had envisioned when I signed up, blood oath and badge in hand, hopeful and brimming with dreams of something better. Now, I was submerged in a nightmare painted with shades of gray and despair, wandering the blurred boundaries between survival and oblivion.

Homelessness wasn't just about lacking a roof overhead or the security of a closed door; it was a brutal stripping away of dignity, identity, and hope—layers of self dissolving in the cold urban wilderness. Each day they passed by, people on their way somewhere, heads fixed ahead, shoulders squared in purposeful strides, while I shrank into the cracked concrete like a ghost no one was obliged to see. I was invisible and glaringly exposed all at once. The world outside marched on, indifferent to the tremors of anguish that rooted me in place, tethered to a cycle of despair. To exist here was a constant negotiation, a precarious balancing act between holding onto remnants of humanity and succumbing to the consuming void that threatened to swallow me whole.

It wasn't always like this. I could still recall, with maddening clarity, the fragments of life before collapse—the echo of voices from a home that no longer felt like mine, the thin line of light in the dingy military barracks where I had clung fiercely to hope, and the cruel fracture when trust shattered amidst brutality. Coming into the military was supposed to be salvation, a fortress against the chaos of the streets I yearned to escape. Instead, it had become another battleground, marking me with scars that no uniform could hide. The sexual violence inflicted upon me had not only violated my body but had dismantled the very foundation of safety and camaraderie I relied upon. My betrayers, cloaked in hatred and cowardice, wielded not only weapons but terror designed to silence me forever. Their threat against my family was a shackle that prevented even the faintest cry for help—a horrific calculus of self-preservation against justice.

In the aftermath, the walls I slammed up around my psyche became both sanctuary and prison. I sought refuge in substances that promised fleeting numbness—a synthetic veil to dull the relentless storm of memories and pain. Alcohol was the first seduction, an old friend that quieted the voices, silenced the screams in my head, if only for a little while. Then the harder drugs crept in, whispering more potent promises of escape, until I was a vessel barely tethered to reality. Addiction was both a curse and a symptom, the merciless twin born from trauma's depths that clawed at my soul with desperate hunger. Days blurred into nights, time losing meaning amidst rituals of use and withdrawal, scavenging for the next hit that might dissolve the ghosts haunting every corner of my mind.

But addiction was only a piece of the fracture. Housing instability wove itself tightly around every aspect of survival. I floated from couch to grimy shelter bed to the cracked cold of city streets, my life a patchwork of profoundly unstable existence. Institutions meant to help often failed or turned away, their doors closed or their hands tied by bureaucracy and stigma. I quickly learned the world saw me as a problem, a cautionary tale, or worse, a disposable soul. Social services were labyrinthine, scattered with red tape and indifferent clerks who barely glanced up when I entered, as if my story were just another statistic lost among the numbers. There was no neat narrative here, only messy, painful chaos that spiraled further the more I tried to grasp control.

Trusting anyone in this wasteland was nearly impossible. The betrayal in the military had rendered me suspicious, defensive, and unwilling to let anyone close enough to see the fractures beneath the surface. I bore the weight of silence, not just from threats but from the deep, paralyzing shame that whispered I was to blame—that somehow the assault, the fall, was my failing. That silence imprisoned me more tightly than any physical chain. Vulnerability meant danger. Seeking help could only invite more harm, rejection, and exposure. So I wrapped myself in invisibility, in shadows and quiet, letting the world pass, a ghost shuttered behind a cracked veneer. Relationships with friends and family frayed under the pressure I surely put on them, the unspoken trauma carving gaps too wide to bridge. Some turned away entirely, fearful, uncertain, or simply tired of the weight. Others tried but stumbled, unprepared for the depth of my hurt or the complexity of my struggle.

Navigating the urban landscape without a steady home was like walking a tightrope over a pit of uncertainty and risk. Every choice—where to sleep, who to trust, how to feed my body and soul—became a calculated gamble with unknown odds. The nights were the hardest, when the city's pulse slowed, and the chaos of survival was stripped bare. Vulnerability increased, predators prowled in shadows, and the cold bit deeper. The overpass under which I found refuge was a cruel irony, an unholy shelter in the form of cracked concrete and graffiti, where rats and restless spirits alike scurried through the darkness. The streets reminded me constantly of the fragility of my existence—a condition easily shattered by one wrong interaction or one careless moment.

Yet, amidst the despair, flickers of resilience fought through. I kept fragments of pride and the shred of will that outweighed surrender. Some mornings, I forced myself to rise from the ground, every joint aching, every thought heavy with doubt, because I remembered who I was—or who I wanted to be. The boy who had escaped gunfire in his neighborhood, the youth who had dared to dream of structure, discipline, and a future beyond the familiar streets. I still carried that spark even when swallowed by darkness, a fragile ember waiting for breath and light. There were occasional moments when a kind word from a stranger or a memory of better times pushed me forward, whispering that I might still find my way.

Psychologically, the trauma embedded itself like an invasive shadow, clouding every thought, coloring every emotion with fear and mistrust. Post-traumatic stress wasn't just a phrase to be thrown around in therapy—it was a tangible, living presence that twisted nerves and pusillanimous hope alike. Memories flashed unbidden—grey faces twisted with hatred, the violent act itself etched in unbearable detail, the cold silence of betrayal echoed endlessly in my mind. Every sound, every touch, every gaze could trigger the floodgates. My body, once a vessel of pride and power, had become a battleground scarred by violation, pushing me into survival mode that was simultaneously hyper-alert and deeply numbed. Sleep was a stranger that favored nightmares, while waking hours crumbled under the weight of recall and repression, a cruel pendulum swinging between extremes. Addiction was the siren's call, the brief promise of peace, but it only pulled me deeper into a vortex of self-destruction.

Intersections of race, trauma, and stigma created a tangled web that further isolated me. As a young African American man, the systemic neglect and racial biases in both civilian and military institutions compounded the barriers to getting help. The very systems meant to protect were often the ones perpetuating silence or minimizing suffering, especially when the victims belonged to marginalized communities. Speaking of sexual assault was labeled weakness or betrayal, and often met with disbelief or outright hostility. The racist undercurrents that stained the military echoed in the neglect and erasure of my pain—a cruel reminder that some lives were less worthy of justice. The legacy of institutional failure loomed large, a cold shadow fostering mistrust that kept wounds festering beneath surfaces too scared or weary to break. My trauma was not viewed in isolation but through the prism of prejudice and systemic indifference. It was a double wound: the physical and emotional trauma inflicted, and the structural betrayal that denied acknowledgment and redress.

Homelessness in this landscape was more than displacement; it was a daily crucible testing will and spirit. Each small victory—finding a safe place to lie down, securing a warm meal, resisting the urge to sink back into addiction—was hard-won and precious. Stability seemed a distant mirage, always just out of reach, no matter how desperately pursued. I was caught in a cycle where the past haunted every step, and the present offered so few firm footholds. Yet, in these depths, I began cultivating a tentative sense of self-awareness—acknowledging the full horror of what had been done to me and the damage wrought over years of displacement. Slowly, painfully, I started to see that survival was not just physical endurance but an act of reclaiming agency where I could.

Despite the shadows, the process of recognizing suffering as trauma rather than personal failure sparked a faint glimmer of possibility. It was the beginning of imagining a different future—a life not defined solely by violence, addiction, and loss, but by healing and reconnection. This recognition, bitter as it was, cracked open the door toward seeking help, even if the path was winding and strewn with obstacles. Finding a therapist who understood, who held space without judgment, was a turning point. The stability that the therapist offered became a scaffold, fragile but real, upon which to rebuild fractured trust. With every session, the fog of numbing substances loosened its grip, anxiety and despair gave way to tentative hope, and the relentless noise of trauma quieted just enough to hear the first seeds of recovery.

The journey from those nights beneath the overpass to standing again as a survivor capable of telling his story was neither linear nor easy. The chaos persisted for a long time, threading through relationships, work, and daily life. Healing was punctuated by setbacks, moments when the past clawed its way back, threatening to undo fragile gains. But the fact that I lived to fight another day was itself a testament to an indomitable, if battered, spirit. Losing ground had meant losing nearly everything I thought I was, only to discover that my identity, perhaps, was not tethered to places or status but to the depths of endurance and the courage to survive the darkest nights.

In those times of homelessness and instability, I grasped the profound complexity of trauma's reach—how violence perpetrated in supposed safe spaces like the military could shatter not just bodies but the very foundations of life. It was not just a personal downfall but a reflection of a system failing its most vulnerable. Understanding this made me see the necessity of advocacy, of breaking silences so no one else would have to fall as far as I did without a lifeline. My story became both a cautionary tale and a beacon of survival, carved out from the darkest experiences to illuminate paths toward justice, healing, and transformation. The streets taught me brutal lessons in pain and resilience, but they also gave me the resolve to reclaim my story from the shadows—and, in doing so, to find the ground beneath my feet once more.

Fractured Relationships

The fractures in my relationships emerged like slow, widening cracks in a fragile glass—almost invisible at first, but over time, so vast and jagged that no gluing or mending could ever truly restore what was lost. Before the trauma, the ties I had with my family and those I cared for carried a certain rhythm, uneven, perhaps, but full of hope and a shared history. Yet, after that night, after the violation and the silencing threat, all those connections that anchored me to a semblance of normalcy began to unravel. It was a gradual disintegration, subtle in moments, devastating in the aggregate, as the tendrils of fear, pain, and shame crept into every interaction I had with the people who once felt like my world.

When I first returned home, the physical wounds hidden beneath my uniform were nothing compared to the invisible ones gnawing at my insides. I carried a silence so heavy it crushed my voice and locked away my truth. In the quiet spaces between words, my family sensed something was wrong, but they could not grasp the full weight of what I was carrying. They saw only the shadows I cast—the distracted glances, the sudden flinches at loud noises, the times I would disappear into myself for hours. My mother's eyes often betrayed her worry, and my father's attempts at tough love fell somewhere between distant and dismissive, fueled by generations of men who believed strength meant stoicism, that vulnerabilities were weaknesses to hide. The cultural and generational chasm widened as I recoiled from their questions, from their mentions of the military as a source of pride and discipline, while inside, I was battling demons they could not see.

Romantic relationships, which might have been a source of solace, became a complex dance of avoidance and misunderstanding. The trauma wounded my ability to trust, undermining the very foundation on which intimacy rests. I would freeze at a touch that should have been comforting, recoiling as if the hands reaching for me were the ones that once hurt me in the most intimate way. The weight of my silence burdened my partners as they sensed my distance but didn't understand the terror behind it. Conversations about futures, about dreams, became impossible as I found myself unable to reconcile my fractured self with the version of a partner they hoped for. Some fled, unwilling to face what they saw as coldness or indifference; others stayed, offering patience but ultimately succumbing to the deep-seated wounds that trauma cements in the psyche. I carried guilt for their pain, and that guilt only built higher walls around my heart.

Family dinners, which once echoed with laughter and clatter of plates, turned into exercises in endurance for everyone involved. The weight of unspoken truths settled over the room like a thick fog. My siblings tiptoed around conversations, uncertain why their brother was no longer the same young man who had once been their biggest protector and confidant. Old friends from the neighborhood drifted away, their own lives winding down different paths or, tragically, succumbing to cycles of violence and addiction that seemed inescapable. I was left in a liminal space, stuck between the world I tried to escape and the one where my nightmares had followed me, engulfing me entirely.

One of the most painful aspects was the unintentional estrangement born from my inability to ask for help. The threat from the men who assaulted me—the explicit warning that my family would suffer if I ever spoke—etched itself deep in my consciousness. That silent promise shackled me in isolation, making it impossible to share the burden of my trauma. My refusal or inability to open up created a chasm of misunderstanding. Relatives interpreted my withdrawal as rebellion or disrespect; they lacked the language, the space, or perhaps the courage to inquire further. I became a ghost haunting my own life, a presence more felt in absence than in action.

In the quiet hours of the night, when the world was asleep, and my thoughts roared loudest, I often found myself replaying memories not just of the assault but of missed moments with those I loved. Birthdays gone uncelebrated, phone calls abandoned mid-conversation, holidays spent alone in motels or on park benches—each a testament to how the trauma dictated my ability to connect. Even when I tried to bridge the gaps, the overlying mistrust made my attempts feel hollow or desperate. The people who once offered warmth recoiled from the coldness that trauma imposed on me, and I recoiled in turn, ashamed of the emotional wreckage I had become.

The addiction that crept into my life was both a symptom and a saboteur of my relationships. It was a cruel echo of the coping mechanisms I believed would dull the relentless pain and silence the intrusive memories. However, as substance dependence took hold, the threads holding me to family and friends stretched further thin and eventually snapped. Loved ones who once stood by me found themselves negotiating the treacherous terrain of co-dependency, disappointment, and heartbreak. Arguments about missed obligations, unexplained disappearances, and broken promises pushed some to the brink of giving up entirely. For those who persisted, their patience was a double-edged sword—marked by genuine concern but also by exhaustion and hurt. I often wondered if they saw me as the person I was before or just the shadow that crumbled beneath the weight of my despair.

There was a persistent, gnawing fear that my trauma would somehow taint or infect everyone I cared about. The idea that my brokenness was contagious forced me further into solitude. I feared that revealing the full story would not only bring harm to my family, as threatened, but also diminish their respect for me. This fear was compounded by layers of shame and the pervasive stigma around male sexual assault, especially in a culture and community marked by rigid expectations of masculinity and strength. I was caught in a prison of silence, the walls constructed from racial trauma, institutional betrayal, and the compounded fears of being misunderstood or dismissed.

Invariably, I found myself confronted with the paradox of needing connection to heal, but feeling incapable of forming or maintaining the very relationships that could offer that healing. It was a vicious cycle: isolation fueled despair, despair fueled self-destruction, and self-destruction pushed people away. I became a stranger to those who had once known me intimately, and worse, I became a stranger to myself. The internal dialogues I carried were raw and relentless. I questioned every interaction, every word exchanged, every lapse in communication. I was haunted by the question of why I deserved such cruelty and whether forgiveness—or even survival—was possible.

It wasn't just personal relationships that fractured; my connection to my own identity dissolved under the first, overwhelming layers of trauma. The boy who had eagerly signed papers to serve his country, seeking a better life and a break from the cycles of poverty and violence, was replaced by a man who felt unworthy, contaminated, and profoundly alienated. These ruptures fed into deep self-loathing and a pervasive sense of being unlovable, which then reinforced the isolation and withdrawal from those around me. The mirror no longer reflected the hopeful youth but rather a haunted figure, weighed down by despair and the threat of future violence.

As time passed, even the people who remained close were affected by multifaceted traumas of their own, including grief over my absence and the painful knowledge that I was carrying heavy burdens alone. The complex dynamics of love and loss played out in every strained phone call, every hesitant visit, every awkward conversation held at a distance. The way I've told it now sometimes barely captures the full dimension of how even well-meaning expressions of concern could feel like judgment or rejection in moments of vulnerability. The subtle undertones of avoidance, the unspoken rules about what could and couldn't be discussed, the ways trauma creates invisible barriers—the cumulative impact was a profound sense of alienation that extended beyond my immediate circle.

Yet amid the wreckage, little moments of grace somehow surfaced. There were family members who refused to let me slip away completely, who, through quiet gestures rather than words, communicated their enduring care and hope for my healing. Some friends from my military days, especially those who had their own scars, reached out with an understanding born from shared suffering. These connections were fragile and often fleeting, but they represented threads of possibility. Even when I couldn't return their trust fully, these gestures reminded me that I was not entirely defined by my trauma and that connection, however complicated, remained vital.

It wasn't until I began the grueling work of therapy that I slowly started to unravel the dense web of pain and shame that had permeated every relationship I held dear. The process demanded that I confront not only my own trauma but the impact it had on those around me. Therapy helped me understand that my reactions—my withdrawal, my anger, my avoidance—were not signs of failure or character flaws, but symptoms of deep psychological wounds. In that recognition came the first fragile seeds of forgiveness, both for myself and, eventually, for those who struggled to understand what I was going through.

With that new clarity, I started reaching out tentatively, rebuilding bridges one stone at a time. It was a slow and uneven process, marked by setbacks and moments of despair, but also by breakthroughs and the reclaiming of trust. I learned to communicate my pain in ways that others could hear without fear, to accept support without shame, and to hold space for the messy, difficult work that healing demands in all relationships. The journey toward restoring fractured relationships was not linear or easy, but it was a vital part of reclaiming my life from the grip of trauma.

Looking back, the breakdown of my family and romantic connections was not merely a byproduct of the assault; it was a reflection of how deeply trauma can permeate every layer of human experience. It illuminated the painful realities of silence and stigma, the intersections of race and masculinity, and the failures of institutions that were supposed to protect, not betray. But it also showed me the resilience buried within, the strength needed not just to survive but to seek restoration—in myself and in those I loved. The fractures remain, some healed, some still tender, but they tell a story of pain, loss, and, ultimately, the unyielding human desire to reconnect and be whole again.

Chapter 6
The Breaking Point

Rock Bottom

The night was thick with cold, as if the air itself conspired to suffocate every flicker of warmth I once clung to. I had found myself perched on the cold concrete steps of a forgotten alleyway, the only sound the distant hum of sirens and the occasional drip of water leaking from a cracked pipe nearby. The city, so alive and unforgiving by day, folded into a quiet cruelty after dark, exposing the rawness of my shattered existence. My body trembled—not from the chill—but from the weight of everything I could no longer bear: the scars etched not on my skin but carved deep within my soul. It was in that frozen night, stripped of all pretense, that I faced the brutally honest truth: I was at rock bottom.

This wasn't a sudden plunge; it had been a slow, grinding descent punctuated by moments of fleeting numbness and bursts of rampant despair. I had been running for years—from gang violence that had stalked my neighborhood like a shadow too large to outrun, from poverty that clawed at my gut every single day, from a crack epidemic that swallowed friends and family alike whole, leaving behind nothing but hollow eyes and broken promises. I ran not just physically but mentally, convinced that the military would be my escape hatch, my salvation. A place where honor, discipline, and brotherhood would shield me from the chaos that had suffocated my adolescence. But the sanctuary I sought held its own horrors, darker than any street corner, more insidious than any gunshot's echo.

The assault—the vile, unforgivable act of violence inflicted by men sworn to protect, men who wore their hate like a badge of twisted pride—shattered whatever hope I had left. Not only was my body violated brutally and mercilessly, but my spirit was broken in ways I could never unwrite or explain without the bluntness of raw pain. Every day after that assault, I carried an invisible weight that crushed my voice, muffled my cries, and twisted my sense of self into unrecognizable knots of shame, fear, and rage. I descended into addiction, as if drowning my anguish in a chemical haze could erase what happened, blur the vivid nightmares that played out behind my closed eyelids, and silence the relentless torment of betrayal.

That night on the cold concrete was, in many ways, just another bleak moment in a long string of nights where I had surrendered to the bottle, to the pills, to the poisonous relationships that only mirrored the violence in me. But tonight felt different—it was as if the walls around me had finally collapsed, and there was nowhere left to hide from myself. The accumulated weight of everything—racism, poverty, assault, addiction, alienation—pressed down with such ferocity that I could no longer breathe. There was nothing left to lose and, paradoxically, nothing left to fight for either. When I looked into the murky puddle beside my feet, distorted by the flicker of a dying street lamp, I barely recognized the reflection staring back—a young Black man, battered beyond belief, whose eyes held a storm of grief and a flicker of a desperate plea for mercy.

Despair clawed at me with teeth sharper than any I'd known, threatening to drag me into a bottomless pit. The idea of giving up was seductive; giving in to the dark promise of oblivion felt like an escape from a life that had turned into a relentless nightmare. Thoughts that were once whispers grew louder—destructive urgencies wrapped in a deceptive cloak of relief. But then, somewhere deep inside the wreckage, a fragile ember of defiance sparked to life. Not because I believed I deserved anything better—that part of me was buried too deeply—but because I realized that surrendering entirely would mean becoming the exact thing that had tried to destroy me: voiceless, invisible, broken beyond repair.

In the quiet and brutal solitude of that moment, I remembered my mother's words from years prior, before the military dreams, before the assault: "You are worth fighting for, even when the world says otherwise." Memories of family dinners, tentative smiles from old friends, the laughter of a child still echoed faintly in my ruined heart. Despite everything, there was a part of me that had not been fully extinguished. That night, sitting alone and drenched in cold shame and disbelief, I made a silent vow—not to erase the past, but to reclaim the shattered pieces of my life. I didn't know how, or if it was even possible, but there was a flicker of something new—a seed of hope buried beneath layers of pain and devastation.

The first flickers of resolve were fragile and coated in fear. Reaching out felt impossible. How could I open the floodgates of my darkest memories without crumbling completely? How could I trust anyone again, after the betrayal cut so deep by those who were supposed to uphold honor and protect? Yet as the night crawled toward dawn, and the city's heartbreak murmured softly around me, I realized that hiding wasn't an option. Addiction and isolation had only deepened the wounds; healing would demand more than avoidance or numbness. I needed help—not just a patch or a temporary fix, but real support from people who understood, who could walk beside me through the shadows rather than turning away.

The next morning, fueled by that fragile decision, I staggered toward a community center where volunteers offered outreach to homeless veterans. My pride was a raw wound; every step was a battle against the shame that threatened to paralyze me. Inside, the fluorescent lights were harsh, and the air smelled faintly of disinfectant and stale coffee, but it was alive with quiet hope. The presence of others who bore scars of their own, who had survived their battles in different ways, eased some of the weight I'd carried alone. For the first time in a long time, I spoke—haltingly at first—about my pain, my fear, my need for more than just survival. The words trembled on my lips, but with each syllable, a piece of the burden lifted, as if the mere act of confession could crack the walls built around my suffering.

From that moment forward, the path toward recovery was anything but straightforward. It was filled with setbacks and self-doubt, moments where the old demons clawed back with desperate ferocity. But the realization I had arrived at in that cold, crushing night sustained me: I would fight for life beyond the darkness—even if the battle was long and the terrain treacherous. Seeking support from the VA, connecting with a compassionate therapist who introduced me to Cognitive Processing Therapy, and finding a tentative anchor in medication and structured treatment became the lifelines I clutched in a sea of uncertainty. They offered me tools to confront the trauma that had imprisoned me, to wrestle with the anger and grief that threatened to consume everything.

That defining moment of hitting rock bottom was not the end of my story but the painful, pivotal point from which true transformation began. It was the brutal acknowledgment that change was essential, and that surviving meant more than merely existing; it demanded courage to rewrite my narrative beyond victimhood. Despite the scars that would always remain, I chose to believe that healing was possible—that my past would not dictate my future. And in that choice, fragile though it was, lay the first glimmer of redemption in the midst of betrayal.

Reaching Out

The moment I realized I couldn't go on like that was neither sudden nor cinematic; it was subtle, creeping like a slow poison that had been coursing through me unnoticed until one day, I just felt utterly empty—an abyss dark enough to swallow every ounce of hope I had left. For years, the numbness and the pain had been locked in a vicious battle inside me—each craving to dominate the fragile hold I maintained on reality. The betrayals, the scars, the whispered threats that once echoed in the brutal confines of the barracks continued to haunt me relentlessly, invading every crevice of my mind and disrupting my life, relentlessly persistent like a chronic storm. When I'd first left home, I had dreamed of a refuge in the military, a place with order, discipline, and an unspoken fraternity that promised safety and respect. Instead, I found myself trapped in a nightmare that obliterated that fragile dream and left me fighting for survival long after I was discharged.

The years that followed the assault were marked by a spiraling descent into addiction and homelessness, each day blending into the next with little distinction but immense suffering. The streets became my grim sanctuary where the bottle was my false friend; it didn't ask questions or demand honesty. It was easier to disappear in intoxication than admit to the roiling chaos inside, the shame that suffocated me whenever I came close to a mirror or reached out for help. Relationships came and went, fractured and broken, unable to withstand the weight of the secret I carried—one that had poisoned my trust, distorted my self-worth, and silenced my voice. It seemed the military's failure to protect me was compounded by my own failure to protect myself from the aftermath, and the silence around my trauma enforced a solitude so absolute that the thought of recovery seemed more distant than ever.

Yet, beneath that paralyzing despair, a fragile thread of hope stubbornly persisted. It surfaced quietly, a faint whisper amid the chaos, a persistent intuition that life could be different. But hope alone was not enough; it needed a catalyst. The turning point came on an unremarkable evening when exhaustion overwrote numbness. I sat alone in a dingy shelter, the night pressing cold against the thin walls, my mind ravaged by memories and dread. In a rare moment, I allowed myself the painful honesty that maybe the endless pain didn't have to be the rest of my story. Maybe, just maybe, there was a way out—but only if I was willing to face the terrifying uncertainty of asking for help.

It was not a decision made lightly. Reaching out meant peeling back the layers I had so carefully built to protect my raw wounds—from the oppressively ingrained mistrust of a system that had failed me and from the fear of exposure, reprisal, and stigma. The military, which I once saw as salvation, had been the source of my deepest betrayal. Was there even a place within those same ranks for someone like me to heal? Was it safe to trust what I had been conditioned to fear? The very thought was fraught with anxiety and the painful memory of what I had endured. Yet, despite every shadow of doubt, I knew I had to try. Living as a prisoner to silence and shame was no longer sustainable; the stakes were too high. Something inside me, perhaps the remnants of the hope I once held as a teenager, pushed me forward toward reclaiming some semblance of peace.

The decision to contact the Veterans Affairs system came with a mix of dread and cautious optimism. I remembered hearing about VA in fragments over the years—the veterans I met along the street sometimes spoke of services, benefits, and counseling, but those conversations were often casual and clouded by suspicion or frustration about bureaucratic hurdles. I had never trusted that place to be a refuge for someone like me, especially given how the military's racial and systemic failures had compounded my trauma. Still, I started researching quietly, using sparse internet access from a public library, piecing together websites and forums for veterans who had endured sexual trauma, trying to find any hint of hope or validation. It was like stepping into a shadowy room, unsure whether I would find a flicker of light or be swallowed by cold darkness.

The initial phone call was a trembling exercise in courage. My hands shook as I dialed the number, each ring echoing with the unspoken fear of rejection or disbelief. When a voice finally answered, calm and professional, I struggled to find the words, fearing that my truth might be dismissed or worse, exploited. But the person on the other end of the line responded with quiet reassurance, guiding me gently through the eligibility process, listening without judgment, and explaining how the VA offered counseling services specifically targeted to Military Sexual Trauma survivors. That moment was a turning tide—a lifeline extended in a sea where I'd felt abandoned. For the first time in years, vulnerability became a precursor to strength, not weakness.

The next step was setting an appointment with a therapist—an idea that was at once terrifying and strangely liberating. I grappled with the anxiety of confronting my trauma head-on, the fear of reliving moments I had buried deep within, and the social stigma attached to mental health in military cultures, especially as a Black man navigating layers of systemic racism and silence. Would the therapist believe me? Could I trust this stranger with the darkest part of myself? These questions haunted me on the days leading up to the session. And yet, beneath the layers of dread, I sensed a small ember of relief—finally, someone willing to see me not as broken or lost but as a survivor worthy of support.

Walking into the VA clinic that day was like stepping into an unfamiliar world, simultaneously clinical and compassionate. The sterile walls seemed less intimidating as the therapist greeted me with warmth and genuine concern, not pity or skepticism. Our first conversations were halting, filled with silence and swallowed words, the weight of all those years of unspoken pain hanging heavy in the room. But, gradually, a fragile bond took root through careful listening and validation, something I hadn't felt in a long time. The therapist introduced me to Cognitive Processing Therapy (CPT), explaining how it focused on understanding and transforming the thoughts and beliefs that trauma imprinted on my mind. The clarity with which they described this path to healing was revolutionary for me—it wasn't about erasing the past but learning to live with it without letting pain dictate every step.

Complementing the therapy, the recommendation to try medication was met with cautious openness. The idea of medication to manage the anxiety, depression, and panic that had long been my constant companions was daunting but promising. Through the combined efforts of therapy and medication, it seemed there was a tangible, hopeful way out of the suffocating cycle of trauma responses that had ruled my life. This integrated approach honored both the emotional and physical realities of recovery, acknowledging that healing is neither quick nor linear but a persistent, courageous journey.

Reaching out to the VA and that therapist shattered the last walls of isolation I had built around myself. It marked the beginning of reclaiming my story—no longer as a victim silenced by fear, but as a man determined to recover dignity and agency. Each session peeled back layers of self-blame and shame, allowed me to speak truths I once locked away, and to confront the deeply rooted pain of betrayal with newfound resilience. The journey was fraught with setbacks and tears, but it was punctuated also by moments of profound insight, gratitude, and the rekindling of hope.

This initial act of reaching out was more than a call for help; it was a rebellion against the silence imposed by trauma and the systemic failures that enabled it. Through this courageous step, I began weaving myself back into the fabric of my own life—one where healing, advocacy, and identity could coexist beyond the shadows of betrayal. And in that emergence, I found not only a path toward recovery but also a calling to break the silence and stigma that too many survivors endure alone. The journey was far from over, but reaching out was the critical first step toward the life I deserved.

First Steps to Healing

The day I first walked into the Veterans Affairs clinic, I was swallowed by an overwhelming mix of dread, skepticism, and a fragile thread of hope that I hardly dared to acknowledge. The sterile scent of antiseptic hung in the air, mingling awkwardly with the low murmur of hushed conversations and the quiet shuffle of feet on cold linoleum floors. I felt like an impostor in this unfamiliar place, a broken young man carrying a lifetime of invisible wounds that no uniform could shield. My hands trembled slightly as I clutched the worn folder that held my medical history—a record fractured by instability, pain, and years of silence. It was my first step toward healing, though at the time, it felt more like stepping into an abyss, unwilling to fully trust that anyone here could truly see the damage hidden behind my stoic mask. The therapist who would become my lifeline greeted me with a calm, steady presence, her voice gentle yet confident, as if to declare, without words, that I was not alone anymore. In that moment, the guarded walls I had erected around myself began to quake, just enough to let in a sliver of light.

At first, the sessions were a blur, loaded with raw emotions I had suppressed longer than I cared to admit. Opening up about the assault—the vivid nightmare of that violent night, the terrifying faces of those men, the sharp sting of betrayal etched into my very bones— felt like exposing my soul to a freezing wind. I coughed up memories that my mind had desperately locked away, memories that clawed at me with sharpened talons. But despite the pain, my therapist's presence was unwavering, her empathetic eyes steady and warm, offering refuge in a storm I was just beginning to navigate. I wasn't just recounting the trauma; I was reclaiming the words that had been stolen from me, piecing together a story that I thought I'd never have the courage to tell. With every session, the crushing weight started to shift, albeit slowly, as I realized that this wasn't about wallowing in darkness but about charting a path out of it. Her belief in my resilience, spoken quietly yet powerfully, became a beacon I clung to in the depths of my despair.

The introduction of Cognitive Processing Therapy, or CPT as she called it, was unlike anything I expected. It was more than just talking; it was a structured journey into understanding how the trauma had distorted my thoughts, shredded my self-image, and poisoned my relationships. Initially, I struggled with the exercises, feeling exposed and vulnerable as I dissected my memories and challenged entrenched beliefs that I was weak or to blame. CPT forced me to confront the demon refusing to let go, but it also handed me tools to fight back, to rewrite the narrative that had defined me for so long. For the first time, I glimpsed a future where I could separate the horrific events inflicted upon me from who I really was—beyond victimhood, beyond pain, beyond shame. Each carefully guided step peeled away layers of guilt and fear, revealing a core of strength that had been there all along, buried beneath the agony.

Medication entered the picture as a companion to therapy, another piece of the complex puzzle of healing. I was hesitant at first, haunted by the stigma surrounding mental health and medicine, but the truth was inescapable: the nightmares, anxiety, and crushing depression weren't going to lift on their own. With measured doses, the fog began to lift ever so slightly, allowing clearer moments of peace and calm where there had only been chaos. The medication didn't erase the pain, but it softened the edges enough for me to engage more fully in therapy and daily life. I started to reclaim the simple joys that trauma had obscured—the warmth of sunlight on my skin, the sound of laughter, the quiet companionship of trusted friends who had stuck by me when I was falling apart. There was a tentative rebirth occurring, pushed along by these intertwined paths of science, empathy, and sheer determination.

There were moments when the waves of self-doubt crashed harder than ever, threatening to undo all the progress. Some nights, the memories surged back with such ferocity that I felt paralyzed, a prisoner to my own mind. Anger, a once suppressed undercurrent, bloomed fiercely—at the assailants, the military system that failed me, and even at myself for surviving in ways I felt ashamed of. Yet the therapy room became a battleground where these emotions could be faced without judgment, a sanctuary where I was allowed to rage, weep, and confront the fragmented pieces of my identity. That space freed me from the suffocating isolation I'd known for so long, reminding me that vulnerability was not weakness but a powerful act of courage. Slowly, I began to replace the silence and secrecy with honest dialogue—not just with my therapist but with myself. The realization that silence had been my prison was painful, but the emerging voice inside me was louder and stronger than ever before.

Hope did not flood in all at once; it was a quiet, persistent ember that flickered in moments I least expected—when I woke from a nightmare and remembered the room where healing was happening, when I smiled at a friend without the weight of anxiety dragging me down, when I could sit still in the light of a new day without the urge to escape. It was the hope that maybe, just maybe, the scars didn't have to define the story of my life. Each small victory—the ability to discuss the trauma without collapsing into despair, the regaining of trust in at least one person, the gradual rebuilding of a sense of self-worth— became milestones marking the arduous climb out of darkness. The therapist's unwavering faith in my capacity to heal became a mirror reflecting the strength I'd long refused to see. For the first time, I was not running from my past but facing it head-on, armed with compassion and tools that offered tangible steps forward.

I also began to grapple with the societal and systemic betrayals that compounded my personal trauma. The thought that four men, bound by a hateful ideology cloaked within the very institution meant to protect, could perpetrate such violence shook me to the core. The threat against my family, intended to silence me, had nearly succeeded, but therapy helped me remember my own power to resist that fear. In those sessions, I found a voice that could speak not only for my own healing but for countless others hidden in the shadows of the military—a voice eager to shatter the silence, confront the racism, and demand accountability. The act of sharing my story became, in itself, a reclaiming of control stolen from me. It was a courageous yet fragile act of defiance against the trauma that sought to keep me broke and bound.

Outside the walls of therapy, I began to rebuild tentative connections with my family and friends. Though the scars remained, the dialogue between us grew richer and more honest. They witnessed a man battling fiercely to reclaim his life, to transform pain into power. This process was neither linear nor easy; setbacks often felt like personal failures, but the compassionate framework provided by therapy served as an anchor. I began to understand that healing was a journey, not a destination, and that resilience was forged through persistence, not perfection. This understanding allowed compassion to seep in—compassion for myself as a survivor, as a human fractured yet made whole through effort and love.

In the mornings after therapy sessions, I often found myself staring out of the window, watching the world beyond—children playing, couples walking, ordinary life in motion. I realized, with quiet gratitude, that I was no longer merely a shadow in this world but an active participant—a man with a story worth telling, a survivor capable of thriving. The first steps toward healing were modest, subtle shifts rather than grand revelations, but they were undeniably profound. Those initial encounters with therapy and medication were not magic cures but the forging of a lifeline. Through connection, understanding, and the hard-won ability to face pain without surrendering to it, these beginnings promised something I hadn't dared hope for before—a future unmarred by silence, illuminated by authenticity, and strengthened by unyielding hope.

Chapter 7
Cognitive Processing Therapy

Understanding CPT

Cognitive Processing Therapy (CPT) arrived in my life like a dim light flickering in a long, suffocating tunnel—tentative but profoundly necessary. What I came to understand first about CPT was that it wasn't simply therapy in the conventional sense, where you talk, and someone listens; it was a rigorous, sometimes grueling journey through the tangled corridors of my own mind. The central principle of CPT is that trauma doesn't just damage our external world; it warps our internal landscape, especially the way we think about ourselves, others, and the future. Those disturbing thoughts and feelings—memories wrapped in shame, guilt, fear, and anger—do not dissolve on their own. Instead, they hold power because of the way they have been interpreted and internalized. CPT challenges and reshapes these "stuck points," those beliefs that chain survivors like me to the wreckage of our past.

Early on, my therapist explained that CPT is grounded in the cognitive model, which asserts that while trauma itself changes reality, it is often the meaning we assign to that trauma that deepens our distress—and this is the very meaning that therapy seeks to transform. My automatic thoughts, those rapid-fire judgments I barely noticed but lived by, were riddled with self-blame and distorted guilt. I believed I was weak, damaged beyond repair, responsible in some twisted way for what had happened to me. This therapy method demanded that I confront those automatic thoughts, analyze their accuracy, and then reframe them with more balanced, realistic perspectives that allow for growth rather than decay.

What made CPT simultaneously daunting and powerful was its structured nature. It was not a vague counseling approach but a step-by-step blueprint that guided me through confronting the trauma head-on, rather than avoiding or numbing it. The initial sessions focused heavily on education, helping me recognize the connection between my thoughts, emotions, and behaviors. I was taught to identify the "impact statements" — my written reflections on how the trauma had affected my beliefs about trust, safety, esteem, intimacy, and control. Writing these down was emotionally wrenching; each sentence peeled back layers of scars I had hidden even from myself. The act of committing these thoughts to paper was both a weight and a release—like carrying chains that suddenly snapped with every word I wrote.

One of the most challenging aspects was the deliberate revisiting of the trauma memory. Unlike other therapies that might favor distancing, CPT asks you to engage with the traumatic event intellectually and emotionally, to dissect the feelings and thoughts it triggers without becoming overwhelmed. This was terrifying at first. Even in the safe room with my therapist, reliving the assault with its vividness scraped open wounds I preferred to keep sealed. Yet, through repeated, guided exposure, the memory lost some of its paralyzing grip. It became a past event rather than a present threat. This process, known as "processing," helped me lessen avoidance behaviors that had kept me trapped in cycles of dissociation and numbing.

Throughout therapy, the challenging cognitive restructuring exercises forced me to wrestle with distorted beliefs such as, "I'm broken," "I am forever unsafe," or "I deserved what happened." Admitting these thoughts felt like admitting failure, which was something ingrained deeply in me from years of survival in harsh environments. However, by carefully questioning the evidence supporting those beliefs and considering alternative explanations, I began to see cracks in those false narratives. For instance, reflecting on the role of the perpetrators illuminated that the betrayal was about their hatred and cruelty, not my worth or actions. Gradually, I recognized how systemic racism and hate, intertwined with sexual violence in the military, had shaped these experiences beyond my control.

CPT's emphasis on the relational impact of trauma was also transformative. The therapy made me acutely aware of how the assault fractured my ability to connect with others—whether soldiers, friends, or family. The fear of being judged, the shame that silenced me, the distrust that isolated me—all these were threads woven tightly around my heart. Through exercises focused on recognizing these patterns, I learned to approach relationships with cautious honesty. It wasn't an immediate fix, but CPT laid the groundwork for rebuilding broken bonds and creating new, healthier connections based on mutual respect and understanding.

There were moments during CPT when I felt as if I was sinking too far under the weight of my own anguish. The cognitive challenges demanded intense introspection and courage that felt exhausting. Some nights, the nightmares persisted as vivid reminders of pain, and the early morning therapy homework seemed impossible. The fear of facing these "sticky points" sometimes led me to resist, to test the boundaries of therapy with silence or avoidance. Yet, my therapist's steady presence and compassionate insistence on persistence made a difference. This journey wasn't about erasing the trauma but transforming my relationship with it—so that it no longer dictated my present and future.

A breakthrough came in a session when I realized I had been carrying the burden not just of the assault but of protecting my family from the threat issued by my assailants. For years, that fear added invisible chains to my suffering: if I spoke out, my family could be hurt. Even after leaving the military, this threat loomed large and deepened my isolation and confession was unthinkable. In therapy, softening this internalized terror allowed me to glimpse a different narrative where I could be safe, and my loved ones could be protected without silence costing me my soul. This realization opened the door to reclaiming my voice, a central goal of CPT.

CPT also addressed the emotional numbness I had developed as a survival mechanism. By guiding me to recognize and label emotions, even painful ones like grief and anger, the therapy encouraged a reconnection with my own humanity. Feeling hurt, sadness, or fear again was not a sign of weakness but proof of healing. The therapy helped me build coping skills to tolerate distress without retreat—skills that were essential to overcoming addiction and homelessness, struggles that had once felt insurmountable.

Another powerful component involved examining the broader social context of my trauma. My therapist brought into conversations the realities of systemic racism and the presence of white supremacist groups like the KKK within the military ranks—factors that had amplified the betrayal and deepened my wounds. Discussing these issues openly within therapy validated my experience and shattered the isolation that comes with believing one is the only victim. It connected my personal narrative to a larger story of injustice, creating a framework for both personal healing and social advocacy.

CPT's homework assignments, which might seem mundane to outsiders, were in fact vital tools of empowerment. Writing impact statements, journaling cognitive exercises, and practicing challenging stuck points forced me to take active ownership of my recovery outside therapy sessions. It wasn't passive or reliant solely on a therapist's words; I had to become the main agent in reclaiming my life and meaning. This responsibility brought with it a sense of control that was paradoxically new and unsettling at first, but eventually liberating.

The progress through CPT was uneven, marked by relapses and moments of doubt. Trauma's imprint is persistent, resisting neat closure or finality. Nevertheless, the therapy laid a foundation for ongoing growth and resilience. It gave me language for my experience and a framework for rebuilding my identity beyond victimhood. It taught me that while pain like mine is deeply personal, it is not isolating—there is a community of survivors who have walked this path and systems being pushed toward reform.

The relationship with my therapist was another indispensable pillar in the process. Her empathy, patience, and unwavering belief in my potential to heal made the hardest moments bearable. She never tried to rush me or diminish my experience but held space for every falter and breakthrough. Her skillful guidance helped me trust the therapeutic process, even when my own defenses screamed to withdraw.

Reflecting back on the entirety of CPT, I realize it was a radical act of self-kindness and rebellion against the forces that had sought to silence and dehumanize me. The cognitive restructuring exercises were not just mental gymnastics but acts of reclaiming my narrative and truth. The time spent unraveling the web of distorted thoughts taught me that while trauma could never be undone, its power to destroy could be diminished and redirected.

Ultimately, Cognitive Processing Therapy planted the seeds for hope in the barren field of my early trauma. It gave me tools to stand tall amidst the wreckage—to recognize that I am not the sum of the worst moments of my life. CPT was the first real step on the long road from betrayal to healing, a painstaking but profound path toward reclaiming trust, dignity, and the promise of a future shaped by courage rather than fear.

Therapy Sessions

Sitting in the muted glow of the small therapy room, the air thick with a mixture of lavender-scented oil and the faint metallic tang of antiseptic, the protagonist felt an odd swirl of unfamiliar emotions. This was not just a room—it was a sacred battle zone where memories long buried, fearful and jagged, would rise and clash against walls of silence he had painstakingly constructed. Each session with the therapist had become a crucible, forcing him into confrontations not only with the raw, gnawing pain of his past but also with his own fragile sense of identity. The therapy began cautiously, almost tentatively, like testing the waters of a dark, expansive ocean. His therapist, a soft-spoken woman with eyes that held an unwavering steadiness, gently introduced him to what she called Cognitive Processing Therapy—a structured approach designed to help survivors untangle the woven threads of trauma, cognition, and emotion. It was strange at first, this expectation to talk openly, to unpack the unbearable. He expected relief; instead, at times, it felt like being dragged underwater, submerged in the suffocating memories of that brutal night in the barracks.

The first few sessions revolved around establishing a thread of trust, a fragile tether between two souls that would gradually be tested and reforged. His therapist did not push him into the abyss immediately but allowed him to navigate at his own bewildering pace, patiently listening to fragmented stories and witnessing his hesitations. She validated each fractured memory, never expressing judgment or impatience, a stark contrast to the military culture he'd fled—a culture that encouraged silence, stoicism, and self-reliance to a fault. Yet as weeks passed, the therapy demanded more than mere recounting; it required him to confront the cognitive distortions nested deep within, those malicious whispers convincing him that the assault was somehow his fault, that vulnerability equated weakness, and that reclaiming his life was an impossibility. He was encouraged to write impact statements, to articulate the meaning of the trauma in his own words. This simple act of expression was agonizing—each sentence a dagger, forcing him to relive the pain, but also paradoxically forging a tentative bridge toward empowerment.

The most harrowing aspect was dismantling the web of shame and self-blame that had engulfed him since the assault. His therapist explained that these feelings were common among survivors, but understanding did little to stem the storm within. On several occasions, the room became a crucible of tears, silence, and broken confessions, his voice cracking as he spoke of the grotesque violation—not just bodily but spiritual—he had endured at the hands of those four men cloaked in both military garb and the vile insignia of hatred. The threat against his family lurked like a shadow, a constant reminder of the dangerous intersection of racial terror and sexual violence. There were days he did not want to come at all, convinced that opening the floodgates of sorrow would drown what little hope remained. Yet, through steadfast presence and gentle encouragement, his therapist helped him navigate the spiral of despair, teaching him grounding techniques—deep breathing, mindfulness exercises—that slowly became weapons against the intrusive waves of flashbacks and panic attacks.

Medication was introduced after a careful psychiatric evaluation, a complementary pillar to the cognitive work underway. Antidepressants and anxiolytics helped stabilize the turbulent sea of his mood, dulling the sharpest edges of anxiety and depression, enabling him to participate more fully in therapy sessions. However, the journey was anything but linear. There were regressions, moments when progress seemed to evaporate, and the dark tendrils of addiction lurked as tempting escapes from unbearable pain. His therapist emphasized the importance of honesty even in these setbacks, fostering a space where relapse was treated not as failure but as part of the complex path toward healing. Some nights, after therapy and medication, sleep still eluded him, haunted by nightmares that replayed the violence in horrifying detail. Yet with time, he began to reclaim his nights, learning to differentiate between memory and present reality, a subtle but crucial victory.

A pivotal breakthrough came several months into therapy, during an exercise designed to challenge the "stuck points" in his thinking. Through painstaking dialogue and written work, he confronted the deeply entrenched belief that the assault had irrevocably destroyed him. Slowly, he began to acknowledge that while the trauma was a part of his story, it did not define his entirety. The sessions in which he vocalized this emerging self-compassion marked turning points, moments when the rawness of pain softened into the tentative possibility of hope. His therapist introduced imagery and visualization techniques, guiding him through scenes of safety and future aspirations, inviting him to imagine a life not ruled by fear and shame. For the first time in years, he dared to dream beyond survival—to envision trust and connection, to imagine relationships not shadowed by trauma.

The therapy also began addressing the complex interplay of his racial identity with the assault, a dimension he had long buried. The fact that his assailants were affiliated with the Ku Klux Klan added layers of terror and hatred to his trauma, entwining it with a historical legacy of racial violence that extended far beyond the military barracks. Processing this racialized dimension was painful yet necessary, as it illuminated the structural failures and silences that had allowed such monstrous acts to fester. His therapist acknowledged the intersectional nature of his suffering, validating the disproportionate impact of MST on Black service members while encouraging him to channel his pain into advocacy and healing. Slowly, the notion of survivor strength began to replace the crushing weight of victimhood.

Therapeutic progress rippled beyond the room, affecting the protagonist's daily life in subtle but profound ways. He began to build tentative bridges with estranged family members, emerging from the shroud of shame that once isolated him. The PTSD that once rendered social interaction impossible gradually receded, replaced by cautious reconnection and renewed empathy. Nights once ruled by insomnia and nightmares grew longer, punctuated by moments of restful peace. The protagonist started to find meaning in small victories—attending social events, practicing self-care rituals, or engaging in community service with veterans who had walked similar paths. Therapy instilled discipline in his fragmented existence, anchoring him with routine and hope.

Yet, the therapeutic journey was not without resistance. There were sessions marked by silence, resentment, and defiance. Sometimes, the protagonist questioned the value of delving so deeply into traumatic pain, fearing that reopening these wounds might only deepen the scars. He wrestled with the pervasive military mentality of toughness, questioning whether vulnerability was a betrayal of the soldier he once aspired to be. His therapist, patient and unwavering, reminded him that healing was not linear and that courage resided not in concealment but in confrontation of pain. This gradual shift transformed therapy from a clinical appointment into a space of authentic dialogue and profound self-discovery.

Over time, the narrative of therapy sessions evolved from one grounded in despair to a story infused with resilience and emerging identity. The protagonist began to write a memoir of sorts within the therapeutic context—a narrative that combined the brutal realities of his MST experience with reflections on survival, race, and the redemptive power of truth-telling. This process, though arduous, helped restructure his belief system, challenging internalized stigma and reclaiming his voice. The act of verbalizing betrayal—not once, but repeatedly—diminished its psychological grasp, transforming it from a source of shame to a catalyst for change.

Another significant aspect of therapy was the incorporation of psychoeducation. The therapist explained the biological and psychological mechanisms underlying trauma, enumerating how the brain rewires itself in response to overwhelming stress and how such changes manifest as hypervigilance, memory suppression, and emotional numbness. This knowledge provided the protagonist with a roadmap to understand his symptoms, alleviating self-judgment by framing his reactions as normal human responses to abnormal events. Realizing that his struggles had a name, a comprehensible framework, empowered him to engage with therapy more actively.

Interspersed throughout the sessions were moments of raw human connection that starkly contrasted with the cold betrayals he had endured earlier. The therapist's unflinching empathy and consistency gradually challenged his skepticism toward authority and support systems. Slowly, he learned to lean into that connection, which nurtured his ability to trust again. He began to share not only his trauma but also his hopes, dreams, and frustrations—a fragile but vital step in rebuilding his shattered sense of self.

The use of homework assignments deepened the therapeutic process. Between sessions, he was encouraged to journal, complete worksheets analyzing his thoughts, or practice relaxation techniques. These tasks, sometimes simple, sometimes emotionally taxing, provided continuity and structure. They forced him to engage with difficult emotions outside the safety of the therapy bubble, cultivating coping skills required for real-world survival. Even when tempted to skip these exercises, the sense of accountability and growing investment in his healing propelled him forward.

At times, the protagonist was haunted by feelings of loneliness and despair that therapy alone could not dispel. It was during those dark hours, he confessed to his therapist, that the opioid and alcohol temptations clawed at his resolve most ferociously. The cycle of addiction was an insidious shadow stalking the edges of his recovery, threatening to undo his gains. The therapist addressed these struggles with sensitivity and pragmatism, connecting him with addiction specialists and support groups. The multidimensional approach, blending trauma treatment with addiction support, reflected an understanding that healing must embrace all facets of his experience.

As therapy unfolded, the protagonist's narrative of self shifted from brokenness to cautious hopefulness. He began to see himself through the lens of resilience—a man scarred but not defeated, defined not by his trauma but by his courage to face it. This new self-concept was fragile, still threatened by waves of doubt and pain, but it was a beginning. The acknowledgment that healing was not about erasing the past but learning to live alongside it became a foundational insight.

The final months of therapy marked a time of integration, where coping skills, emotional regulation, and self-compassion crystallized into daily practice. The protagonist no longer viewed therapy as a separate ordeal but as an extension of his commitment to reclaiming a life once shattered. He began to mentor other survivors, lending his voice to advocacy groups, finding strength in solidarity. The therapy space, once a crucible of terror and despair, had transformed into a platform for rebirth and empowerment.

Throughout the entire therapeutic voyage, the protagonist wrestled continuously with the haunting memories of betrayal, not only personal but institutional—the military's failure to protect and the systemic racism that enabled violence to thrive. Therapy equipped him not just with tools for personal recovery but with a fortified voice to challenge injustice. He emerged not only as a survivor but as an advocate, ready to confront the silence and stigma surrounding Military Sexual Trauma.

In essence, the therapy sessions were not simply treatment; they were an unyielding journey through darkness and light, a dance between despair and hope, a testament to the indomitable human spirit. Each session carved space for truth, pain, grief, and ultimately, healing—a sacred retreat where the protagonist could slowly piece together the broken mosaic of his life and reclaim his story from the shadows of betrayal.

Processing Trauma

Processing trauma was not a linear journey, nor was it the gentle unfolding of neatly packaged memories one could sort through like photographs spread on a table. It was a tumultuous excavation of the self, an excavation that unearthed pain, confusion, anger, shame, and, surprisingly, glimmers of resilience buried deep beneath the rubble of sorrow. Each therapy session with Dr. Calloway felt like stepping into a storm, one that threatened to overwhelm yet promised cleansing in its wake. The process began with a commitment that was as frightening as it was hopeful: to confront the harrowing events that had long been shrouded in silence and denial. At first, I recoiled from the echoes of my past. The memories of that horrific night—four white men, emboldened by racist hatred, violating my body with a mop handle and words as sharp as knives—were etched in my mind's eye with brutal clarity. Their threats were chains that held not only my body but my voice captive, warning that any cry for help would bring devastation upon my family. The weight of that threat had anchored me in silence for years.

Yet, in the quiet room of the VA, surrounded by the soft hum of fluorescent lights and the soothing presence of a therapist who believed in my survival, I made the painful choice to speak. Cognitive Processing Therapy (CPT) was introduced to me not as a magic cure but as a disciplined framework to dismantle the cognitive distortions that trauma had insidiously planted. Initial sessions were excruciating;

I found myself retelling the story over and over, as if by repeating it aloud I might wrest control from the ghosts that haunted me. With every detailed recounting, the fresh wounds seemed to reopen, oozing raw emotion that I'd long tried to bury. Shame surged fiercely, twisting my stomach into knots, insisting I was damaged beyond repair. But Dr. Calloway's gentle persistence and her unwavering insistence that I was not to blame began to chip away at those toxic beliefs. She taught me that trauma lied not in the memories themselves but in the meaning I had assigned to them.

Together, we unraveled narratives that had cemented themselves in my psyche: beliefs of helplessness, worthlessness, and self-blame that had shaped the darkest corners of my existence. I had convinced myself that my enlistment, my dreams of escape and purpose, had been folly, that I had somehow invited punishment for wanting more from life. The essential work of CPT required me to identify these "stuck points" — the cognitive traps where my pain had festered. Mapping these beliefs was like drawing a battlefield blueprinted by fear and prejudice. I confronted ideas that screamed I was weak for surviving, that I was tainted because of what was done to me, and that I was unworthy of love and safety. Each revelation was a drop in the bucket of shadows I had carried alone for so long. The act of articulating these painful thoughts out loud, with a compassionate listener holding space, began to loosen the grip these narratives had on me.

Yet these sessions were not without setbacks. There were days when my body betrayed me: flashbacks would crash over me without warning, drowning my awareness in the violent sensory details of the assault, leaving me gasping for breath in the middle of a conversation or curled in a ball of shame on my bed. These moments of re-experiencing the trauma were harrowing, but with Dr. Calloway's guidance, I learned to ground myself, focusing on physical sensations like feeling my feet press into the floor or the rhythm of my breathing, reminding my mind that I was safe in the present. The pain felt so vivid it seemed to tear apart the fragile membrane separating past from present, but learning to differentiate between then and now was essential in reclaiming my autonomy. The therapist's steady presence was a lifeline; when the nights spiraled into nightmares or the days blurred with numbness, her voice in my ear reminded me that healing was messy, that it didn't demand perfection but resilience.

One of the most difficult aspects of the therapy was processing the betrayal not only of the assault itself but of the institution I had trusted. The military was supposed to be a haven, a brotherhood that would shield me from the chaos I had fled in my neighborhood. Instead, it became the stage for the worst kind of racialized violence, perpetrated by white supremacists disguised in uniform. Exploring this betrayal challenged my very identity. I grappled with anger boiling beneath my skin but also with profound isolation, for how could anyone understand the compound nature of this trauma? Talking about racialized sexual violence in spaces that seemed designed to deny or minimize it felt like wading through a swamp that exhaled poison with every step. Dr. Calloway helped me name these feelings— disillusionment, despair, indignation—and to understand that facing systemic betrayal was as critical as healing my individual wounds. The therapy became a mirror reflecting not just my own brokenness but the fractures in a system that failed to protect me.

After several months, amidst the trials and painful quiet breakthroughs, I reached a moment that felt like a crack of light splitting through an overcast sky. During a particularly raw session, I read aloud a written account of my trauma—no longer muffled, no longer cloaked in shame. As I spoke the words, describing the assault and the threat cast over my family, the weight that had long pressed down on my chest began to lighten. I realized the story no longer owned me; I was reclaiming it, giving it back its rightful place as a wound, not a definition. This breakthrough was not a triumphant exclamation but a quiet acknowledgment of something deeply significant: I had begun to separate my identity from the trauma. It was not who I was, but a chapter in the story I was still writing. This shift marked a turning point that emboldened me to confront other shadows—emotions I had numbed with alcohol, relationships I had sabotaged out of fear, and a future I had long thought impossible.

Therapy also required integrating the use of medication, a tool I initially resisted. The stigma attached to psychiatric prescriptions lingered in my mind like a ghost of old battles, but the medication brought a stabilizing effect that allowed the fog of anxiety and depression to recede enough for my cognitive efforts to gain traction. The combination of medication and CPT was pivotal, each component reinforcing the other, weaving a safety net underneath the often precarious steps of recovery. Side effects tested my patience, with moments of lethargy and blurred focus, but Dr. Calloway's careful monitoring and adjustments affirmed that healing was a process of trial and error, a rehearsal in patience and self-compassion.

Processing trauma was also a confrontation with the false narrative that survivors carry alone—that they are broken, unfixable, and destined to carry the scars in silence. Each session built a counter-narrative that whispered of strength, survival, and the possibility of wholeness. The therapeutic space became a crucible where pain was transformed into insight, and insight into hope. I learned to recognize triggers—an unexpected glance, a phrase, a scent—that could summon the past, and developed strategies to disarm them rather than be defeated by them. I relearned how to trust my instincts and, tentatively, established boundaries in relationships, wary but willing to risk vulnerability again. Trust, once shattered, had seemed an impossible bridge to rebuild, but with time and effort, small bricks of reliability and honesty were laid down upon the ruins.

The most profound challenge was allowing myself to mourn—not just the assault and its immediate consequences, but the erasure of the future I had envisioned. The dreams of service with honor, of pride and brotherhood, were replaced with a dark shadow of betrayal and loneliness. Mourning is a crucible, a necessary burn to clear away what no longer serves, and therapy held space for this grief without judgment. It was in this space that I began to rediscover pieces of myself long thought lost—the young man who had stepped away from a violent street life hopeful for better, who deserved more than the violence he endured. Through this process, healing expanded beyond the individual, touching the interconnected lives of my family and community, because reclaiming my voice echoed into theirs, a quiet call for solidarity and recognition.

Even now, processing trauma remains an ongoing journey rather than a destination. There are days when the weight resurfaces unexpectedly, when memories play like old films in the background of daily life. But the tools acquired through therapy have forged a resilience that allows me to meet these days not with surrender but with mindful presence. The story I tell myself now is not one of victimhood but of survival, not silence but voice, not shame but courage. Processing trauma has meant navigating the terrain of pain with a compass of hope, guided by the belief that even the deepest wounds hold the possibility of transformation, and that through the darkest betrayals, the human spirit can reclaim light.

Chapter 8
Medication and Healing

Prescription Journey

The journey of finding the right medication was anything but straightforward. At first, the very idea of medical intervention felt foreign and uncomfortable. After years of existing under the crushing weight of trauma without adequate support, the protagonist was understandably wary of handing control over any part of himself to another—especially in the form of pills. The room where he first discussed medication with the VA psychiatrist had a sterile chill to it, filled with the low hum of machines and faint echoes of conversations drifting through the thin walls. It felt clinical, detached—a sharp contrast to the raw pain searing his memories. Yet, the compassionate therapist had explained gently that medication could be an ally, a tool to help temper the unbearable tides of anxiety, depression, and intrusive thoughts that had ruled his days and nights. It was a reluctant acceptance, mixed with a fragile hope, that set this chapter of his recovery into motion.

The initial prescription was a modest dose of a selective serotonin reuptake inhibitor, an antidepressant aimed at easing the crushing fog that had settled over his mind. The first few days brought a kind of numbing wave, dulled emotions drifting past like muted whispers, and a curious detachment from the fiery swirl of memories that often erupted without warning. But this also meant a flattening of intensity, including moments of fleeting joy or hope that previously lived in his dreams or the rare comforting memory. Side effects became a constant companion: early mornings greeted him with nausea that twisted his stomach into knots, and a persistent headache settled in his temples like an uninvited guest refusing to leave. His sleep, once fragmented by nightmares and cold sweats, shifted unpredictably—sometimes drifting into deep, dreamless silence, other times plagued by unsettling restlessness that left him more exhausted than before.

The trade-offs weighed heavily on him; the medication dulled the pain but also dulled his sense of self. Friends and the therapist noticed the changes—some good, some worrisome. Conversations became more measured, emotions more contained. The substance of his worries flickered but didn't fully extinguish. A growing tension brewed inside: the desire to be rid of the hauntings without losing the very essence that made him who he was. It was clear that this single medication was only a tentative beginning, not a fix. After several weeks marked by this cautious dance, adjustments were necessary.

The psychiatrist took time reviewing his feedback, carefully listening to the protagonist's descriptions of mood shifts and physical discomfort. It required delicate balancing—a constant weighing of benefits against side effects. The dosage was altered incrementally, experimenting with timing so the sickly nausea could be minimized, taking medicines with food, before bedtime, or splitting doses. But still, his spirit felt stifled. This led to the introduction of a secondary prescription—an anxiolytic, meant to quell the ceaseless storms of anxiety that gripped him tightly in both expected moments and sudden, brutal episodes. It was a bitter pill to swallow, literally and figuratively, surrendering further autonomy and wading deeper into the realm of psychopharmacology, but desperation shaped his choices.

At times, the anxiolytic worked like a balm, smoothing the sharp edges of panic attacks and allowing him to breathe when the weight of past horrors pressed down unbearably. The crushing tightness in his chest loosened marginally, and for certain hours, he experienced an unprecedented calm. Yet, side effects shadowed progress—a sluggishness that hovered at the edges of perception, a clouded mind that sometimes made concentration a distant dream. The transformation wasn't linear; some days brought progress, others retreat. He learned to negotiate with his own body and mind, recognizing that the medicines, in their imperfect nature, could not erase trauma but might build a scaffold that would eventually support healing.

Throughout this process, the protagonist grappled deeply with internalized stigma. Medication was often perceived as a weakness in the military culture he had tried so hard to embrace—admitting need for help equated to vulnerability, or worse, failure. These internal barriers complicated his relationship with treatment. But the growing trust in his therapist's steady presence and gentle reassurance transformed his willingness. The therapist framed medication as a form of empowerment, a way of reclaiming control from the wreckage of trauma rather than surrendering to it. This shift in perspective, subtle but powerful, helped the protagonist embrace the medications as tools in his arsenal rather than chains.

One unexpected challenge emerged from the medications themselves: fluctuations in mood and identity perception. There were moments when the protagonist looked in the mirror and felt like a stranger; the face staring back was the same, but the emotional undercurrents felt alien—muted, disconnected, sometimes eerily numb. It sparked a profound existential discomfort. Who was he if not the raw, tormented soul tangled in the wreckage of his memories? How did he reconcile the medication's effects with the desire for authenticity? Talking these feelings over in therapy helped, but the process was agonizing. The fog of pharmaceuticals blurred lines between survival and numbness, between coping and hiding.

Eventually, the psychiatrist recommended a new medication—this one targeting sleep disturbances more directly, a low-dose hypnotic designed to reestablish healthier rest patterns. Sleep had been a battleground since the assault, a time when nightmarish images hijacked his mind and left him drained. The hypnotic did not erase dreams but helped create space for restorative sleep cycles, enabling his brain to begin the delicate work of processing trauma in more manageable fragments. This brought a subtle but vital shift; increased restful rest fortified his struggling will, and for once, mornings didn't arrive heavy with the weight of exhaustion and despair.

Slowly, the medication regimen morphed into a personalized balance, a carefully calibrated constellation responsive to his unique biology and experiences. No longer was it a blunt instrument but a nuanced support system aiding gradual breakthroughs. Over time, improvements mounted in small but undeniable increments: anxiety less ensnaring, intrusive memories less paralyzing, moods less volatile, and core resilience steadily re-emerging from beneath layers of pain and coping mechanisms. The medications never became a cloak to hide behind but a scaffold on which he could rebuild fragments of self.

Complementing the pharmacological journey was his increasing understanding of side effects—not as failures but as parts of the process requiring patient attention and adjustment. Some days were harder, tougher to balance; others were triumphs of endurance and small victories. He learned the importance of self-monitoring, keeping journals of moods and symptoms, and maintaining open dialogue with his healthcare providers. This partnership formed a vital lifeline, replacing the isolation his trauma once imposed.

Medication also played a critical role in breaking down some of the defenses that trauma had built around his mind and heart. As the storm within gained moments of calm, he could engage more deeply in cognitive processing therapy, confronting painful memories with a renewed clarity and less paralyzing fear. The combined benefits of therapy and medication work created synergistic momentum, slowly shifting his narrative from one of helpless victimhood toward empowerment.

But the journey remained fraught. At times, it was difficult to distinguish medication-driven mood shifts from the residues of trauma. The grasp of memories could still overwhelm him, even with the pharmacological support. The challenge was persistent: to remain vigilant and adaptive, recognizing that healing was not a destination but an ongoing process with setbacks and triumphs alike. The protagonist embraced this reality with growing maturity shaped by experience and guided compassion.

Throughout the prescription journey, a broader revelation unfolded about systemic failures. The difficulty in accessing appropriate medications, the trial-and-error approach common in psychiatric medicine, and the stigma surrounding mental health treatment in military and African American communities all became painfully evident. Navigating these waters required resilience beyond mere survival—demanding self-advocacy and sometimes pushing back against institutional inertia. His story illuminated how critical it was to dismantle these barriers for future survivors who deserved timely, culturally sensitive, and effective treatment.

By chronicling this medication journey, the protagonist not only tracked his steps toward recovery but began to reclaim a narrative of agency and strength. Each adjustment, every new pill introduced or discontinued, became a symbol of his refusal to be silenced or broken. The medicine was never a panacea but an essential part of a mosaic that was his healing process, affirming that recovery, though complex and hard-fought, was within reach.

In retrospect, the protagonist recognized that medication was not a simple escape from pain but a bridge through it—a means to endure, confront, and ultimately transform. The physical sensations of side effects faded into the background as the emotional healing gained ground. Through this ongoing prescription journey, he reclaimed aspects of his life stolen by the assault, rediscovered shades of hope dimmed by years of darkness, and laid the foundation for a future where trauma no longer defined him.

Managing Side Effects

Navigating the labyrinth of medications was, for him, a journey fraught with contradictions—relief shadowed by new burdens, hope tangled with unexpected hurdles. At first, the prospect of medical intervention, of something tangible to battle the relentless torment in his mind, offered a fragile glimmer of solace. The therapist had carefully explained the regimen: a combination of antidepressants and anxiolytics, small doses cautiously introduced to stabilize the storm beneath his skin. Yet, as days bled into weeks, what began as a promise wrestled stubbornly with harsh realities. Alongside the gradual easing of raw, searing anxiety and the numbing waves of depression, unwelcome companions—side effects—anchored themselves deeply in his daily existence, testing his resolve with every breath.

The mornings started with fog, a sluggish descent into consciousness that dulled not only the pain but his clarity and energy. His body moved through rituals mechanically, weighed down by a persistent lethargy that no caffeine or sheer willpower could undo. Tasks that once seemed simple, like rising from bed or brushing his teeth, became mountainous endeavors requiring mental negotiation, as if his muscles had forgotten their purpose. This cumbersome drowsiness hung over him like an oppressive shroud during training sessions and therapy appointments alike, often prompting a haunting question: was this sedation part of healing or merely another form of imprisonment? There were days when the medication's sedative grip became so overwhelming that it felt as if he were trapped inside his own body, disconnected from the urgent pulse of life that surged beyond his window.

Alongside fatigue, a creeping numbness inserted itself between him and the world, dulling the sharp edges of trauma but also muting moments of joy, triumph, and human connection. The vibrant colors of everyday life receded into muted grays, turning laughter and love into distant echoes. While the tormenting flashbacks and nightmares softened in intensity, the price was an emotional flatness that unsettled him profoundly. He mourned the erosion of spontaneity and the dimming of passion—elements that once defined his identity before the assault ruptured his course. The very chemical agents intended to restore balance paradoxically stripped away his capacity to feel fully alive. Each day became a negotiation between the desire for relief and the fear of losing the essence of who he was beneath the therapeutic haze.

Physical discomfort manifested insidiously, as shifting weights in the stomach, waves of nausea that stole his appetite, and a restless agitation that surged unpredictably through his limbs. Nights were often consumed by an innate restlessness that medications seemed unable to quell, twisting his sleep cycles into fractured patterns of fitful wakefulness and unrestful slumber. The battle that had begun within his mind now echoed viciously through his body, reminding him that recovery was neither linear nor gentle. Sometimes, the trembling fingers and tightening chest became so pronounced that he questioned whether it was the trauma revisiting him or the drugs waging their own quiet war inside. These conflicting sensations blurred boundaries, fostering a deep sense of confusion and exhaustion that compounded his vulnerability.

Compounding these difficulties was the delicate balancing act of dosage adjustments. His therapist and psychiatrist approached his treatment with cautious optimism but recognized the individual's complex biochemical responses. Incremental increases in medication could bring improved symptom control but risked intensifying side effects, while decreases offered relief from physical discomfort at the potential cost of mental clarity. He found himself living in a state of uneasy equilibrium, where every change threatened to upset the fragile progress painstakingly achieved. Days of hope could quickly be undermined by new waves of dizziness, disorientation, or emotional volatility, leaving him feeling as if he were trapped within an unpredictable vortex. The necessity of transparent communication with his healthcare providers became paramount, yet at times, the stigma of mental illness and past trauma complicated these vital dialogues, engulfing him in a private battle of trust and courage.

Family interventions underscored this complex picture—his mother's worried glances and tentative questions revealing both her concern and her limited understanding of psychiatric medication's intricacies. Their conversations sometimes drifted into frustration, with him caught between his desire to explain and the inexplicable nature of side effects that words could only partially convey. His siblings, though supportive, occasionally reacted to the sudden changes in his demeanor with mistaken assumptions of laziness or indifference. The social ripples of medication challenges underscored another painful reality of trauma recovery: healing was rarely a solitary path but entwined with the perceptions, hopes, and fears of loved ones wrestling alongside him. Yet, despite these challenges, the steady presence of the therapeutic team remained a beacon, their empathetic insistence that adjustments were a natural part of the healing journey easing some of the isolation that medicine's side effects sometimes imposed.

Adjusting to medication was also a psychological confrontation with control—or rather, the loss of it. Having lived under the weight of betrayal, manipulation, and threats, surrendering to a regimented pharmaceutical schedule was rife with ambivalence. He grappled with the fear that his vulnerabilities could be further exploited, that dependence on pills might erode his agency just as trauma had diminished his trust. This internal conflict was compounded by occasional flare-ups of paranoia and distrust towards the very system meant to support him. Yet, grounding himself in the therapist's patient explanations and clinical care slowly rebalanced these fears, allowing him to view medication not as a crutch but as a vital tool in reclaiming autonomy over his fractured mind and body. Such realizations, painful as they were to acquire, became pivotal moments that nurtured deeper engagement with his treatment plan and a rekindled belief in his capacity to heal.

Over time, subtle yet meaningful improvements emerged, sewing threads of hope through the fabric of his daily life. The thunderous nightmares lessened in frequency and intensity, their aftermath no longer leaving him paralyzed in bed, drenched in cold sweat and suffocated by dread. Mornings, though still often slow and dull, gradually gained a sliver of sharpness—the kind that nudged him towards purposeful actions rather than mere survival. His thoughts, once littered with relentless self-blame and despair, began to organize, enabling him to reengage with therapy sessions more constructively. Medication, imperfect and demanding constant negotiation, nonetheless became a gateway to this functional clarity. Even the hardest days carried within them fragments of possibility, the fragile proof that recovery was neither myth nor distant dream but a strenuous, multifaceted process he was slowly mastering.

The interplay of side effects also prompted him to develop an acute self-awareness and self-compassion previously foreign to his experience. He learned to monitor his body's signals attentively—recognizing when fatigue signaled the need for rest rather than weakness, understanding that nausea might resolve with dietary adjustments, and that emotional blunting required honest conversations with his therapist. This attentive stewardship of his well-being became a new form of resilience, a dynamic dialogue between mind and body rather than a passive acceptance of pharmaceutical consequences. It was an empowerment born not from the absence of suffering, but from the courageous navigation of its complexities and continuities. Through this process, the rigid boundaries that trauma had imposed began to soften, replaced by a fluidity that allowed for struggle and recovery to coexist.

Medication side effects also interlaced with his broader social and occupational reengagement. Returning to community life after periods of isolation was riddled with practical challenges—attending appointments required managing dizziness and fatigue; reconnecting with old friends necessitated patience in facing moments of emotional disconnect; reentering the workforce demanded an accommodation of fluctuating mental and physical stamina. Employers and peers, not always aware or sensitive to invisible illnesses, sometimes dismissed his struggles or misattributed them to a lack of motivation. This external skepticism reinforced painful stigmas, compounding the internal battles fostered by medication-induced changes. Yet, these challenges also galvanized advocacy and education efforts in his recovery journey, motivating him to become a voice not only for survivors of trauma but for the often undermined realities of those healing amidst the shadows of side effects.

There were moments, stark and unforgiving, when the perseverance required felt almost unbearable. Times when nausea would force him to spend hours curled on the floor, or the fog of sedation blurred the line between night and day, wrenching away his sense of rhythm and grounding. The seeming permanence of these afflictions sometimes threatened to eclipse the gains made, tempting despair and withdrawal. But woven through these darkest hours was an emerging narrative of endurance shaped by small victories: a morning woke without dread, a day completed at work, a therapy session attended with clarity—each an act of rebellion against the silent tyranny of trauma and its medicinal counterparts. His will, though battered, remained unbroken, anchored in an evolving conviction that healing was an imperfect, ongoing process demanding kindness as much as determination.

The labyrinth of managing medication side effects was, ultimately, a crucible reshaping the contours of his identity and resilience. It was a stark reminder that recovery from the wreckage of trauma was neither quick nor neat, but a tangled passage through shadow and light. The medications themselves were not villains nor saviors but complex agents within a broader tapestry of survival, therapy, human connection, and self-awareness. By embracing the fluidity of this journey, by facing discomfort and uncertainty with an open heart, he cultivated a deeper understanding of what it meant to reclaim his life—not as a victim defined by betrayal, but as a survivor armed with knowledge, patience, and fierce hope.

Positive Changes

The first inkling of true change came gradually, like the slow dawn creeping over a long, dark night that had seemed endless. For years, the protagonist had drifted through existence battered by the rough seas of trauma, addiction, and loneliness, a ghost haunting his own life. His mind was a battlefield where memories crashed relentlessly, and his spirit bore the jagged scars of betrayal and violence that had no easy balm. When he first walked into the VA facility, the sterile whiteness of the walls and the steady hum of fluorescent lights felt alien, cold, a sharp contrast to the chaos that had marked every step of his journey. Yet, it was within those walls, under the guidance of a therapist who saw through his guarded exterior, that the first threads of a new narrative began to form—one not dictated by pain and fear, but slowly woven with strands of hope and possibility.

The introduction to medical intervention marked a turning point. At first, the mention of medication sparked a cocktail of skepticism and fear. There was a lingering mistrust seeded by years of neglect— not only by the institution but by his own body that had betrayed him by succumbing to nightmares, panic attacks, and unbearable flashbacks. The pills were presented not as a magic cure but as a tool—part of a comprehensive approach designed to steady the tumultuous waves of his mental health struggles. Antidepressants and anxiolytics entered into his daily routine carefully, with close monitoring and adjustments that gave him a sense of control for the first time in years. Side effects were challenging at times: moments of fatigue that made even simple tasks daunting, occasional bouts of nausea that reminded him the cure was a process rather than a gentle fix. But these hurdles became small blips against the larger constellation of newfound clarity.

Perhaps the most profound shift was not just in the lessening of symptoms but in the burgeoning sense of normalcy in everyday functioning. Where once waking up was a daily confrontation with despair, mornings began to hold small promises. The fog that clouded his mind—the relentless swirl of intrusive thoughts and an unending current of fear—began to lift, or at least thin, enough so that he could distinguish memories from present reality without drowning in pain. The mental lethargy that had rendered him a prisoner of his own trauma loosened its grip, allowing him to plan, to dream, and to engage with life outside the perpetual shadow of his darkest moments.

Therapy sessions with his compassionate therapist were a cornerstone of this transformation. Cognitive Processing Therapy (CPT) was rigorous and unrelenting in its honesty but framed in a way that respected his pace, his limits. It was within the safe confines of these sessions that he confronted the tangled web of beliefs that trauma had knotted inside him. The pervasive, poisonous narrative of self-blame, the suffocating silence forced by fear of retribution, and the deep wounds infused by racism and hate—the therapist helped him dismantle these lies piece by piece. Not by erasing pain, but by recontextualizing it, allowing him to reclaim power over his own story. Each session was a grueling excavation, sometimes dredging up memories that made his heart pound with fear and shame, but always ending with a sense of emerging into light.

With each week, therapy became less about surviving and more about healing. He learned skills to soothe the storm within—a blend of mindfulness and grounding techniques that tethered him to the present, safety, and control. The nightmares diminished in frequency as he harnessed strategies to challenge the intrusive images that once ruled his nights. Anxiety no longer dictated his every breath; it became a visitor, a shadow that could be acknowledged and gently, firmly sent away. Gradually, his thoughts about himself shifted—the loathing and self-reproach replaced by cautious self-compassion. The idea that he was not defined by the brutality he endured, but by his strength to face it, began to take root. This evolving mindset was as crucial as any medication, a silent revolution within his psyche.

Improvements in mental stability rippled outward into the practicalities of daily living. Tasks that once felt insurmountable—the simple acts of eating regularly, maintaining hygiene, or managing his living environment—became attainable goals rather than insurmountable barriers. Structure returned to his day, something that had proved elusive when addiction and despair held sway. The fog of addiction that had blurred the edges of his reality began to lift, aided not only by therapy and medication but also by the reestablishment of routine and community. Support groups at the VA introduced him to peers who had navigated similar battles, offering solidarity and the powerful realization that he was not alone. Their stories intertwined with his, weaving a sense of belonging that past rejection and isolation had denied him.

Physically, his health also improved as the mental chaos settled. The body, long neglected and abused as a vessel of pain and shame, responded to the slowing of psychological torment. Regular sleep patterns took hold, and with rest came renewed energy and a rebuilt immune system. He could hold conversations without being overwhelmed by flashbacks. The aches and tension that had been constant companions lessened, indicating that healing was extending beyond the realm of the invisible wounds. His appearance, once marked by neglect and the wear of survival on the streets, showed signs of care and respect, small victories that radiated self-worth.

Despite progress, the journey was far from linear or smooth. Medication adjustments brought moments of doubt—a day where dizziness made steps uncertain, or mood swings blurred the edge of confidence. There were lapses when the past's shadows threatened to swallow him whole, moments when the weight of silence and secrets bore down anew. But these moments were now tempered by tools and relationships that grounded him, preventing total collapse. Relapses into despair no longer defined the horizon but were viewed as obstacles to be overcome, bumps on the road that demanded patience and resilience.

An unexpected but vital dimension of improvement was the rekindling of relationships. Family, once damaged by the distance and secrecy wrought by trauma, began to rethread their connections. The protagonist's willingness to share parts of his journey—fraught and painful as they were—offered his relatives insight and empathy that had been missing before. Forging honesty in these relationships was not instantaneous nor easy; it required time, repeated attempts, and the rebuilding of trust. Yet, each meaningful interaction restored a sense of grounding in his identity, anchoring him beyond the confines of victimhood and despair. Friendships, both old and new, blossomed as he reclaimed his narrative and found the strength to be vulnerable. The isolation that had been a near-constant companion was slowly replaced by the warmth of human connection.

As confidence in his coping mechanisms grew, the protagonist began to explore activities that once seemed out of reach. Volunteering, attending educational workshops, and engaging in advocacy programs at the VA became not only diversions but purposeful endeavors that enriched his sense of self. These activities fostered pride and offered a tangible way to reclaim agency over his life trajectory. The notion of a future, once blurred by trauma and addiction, sharpened into clearer focus. He envisioned a life not shackled by what had happened but defined by the possibilities of what lay ahead.

The therapeutic alliance with his counselor emerged as a pillar of support, an anchor in the sea of healing. The therapist's nonjudgmental presence, careful listening, and tailored interventions carved a safe space where vulnerability was not punished but embraced. Shared milestones—like confronting previous denial, dismantling self-harmful beliefs, and developing emotional regulation—became markers of progress that buoyed the protagonist's spirit. The therapeutic process was not solely about confronting pain but also about nurturing the capacity for joy, hope, and trust, elements once shattered in the assault and its aftermath. This professional relationship was instrumental in transforming trauma from a life sentence into a surmountable challenge.

One of the most profound internal shifts was the reclamation of self-trust. For so long, the betrayal had seeded doubt about his own perceptions and worth. Relearning to listen to his own voice, respecting his boundaries, and asserting his needs was a subtle but revolutionary act of empowerment. Therapy encouraged him to articulate his experiences on his own terms, turning the silence imposed by threats and fear into liberation through expression. This empowerment radiated outward, affecting daily interactions and long-term goals alike. The internal dialogue changed from one of self-punishment to one of self-advocacy.

Healing also meant confronting the enduring scars of racial violence embedded within the trauma. The protagonist grappled with the complex intersection of race and victimization—the way racial hatred fueled the assault and how systemic racism shaped the military institution's failure to protect him. His recovery involved not only personal restitution but an acute awareness of the broader social and institutional wounds. This dual awakening informed his advocacy work and commitment to fostering change within military and civilian systems alike. He carried the memory of his trauma as both a burden and a beacon, illuminating the urgent need for transparency, accountability, and reform.

As time progressed, the protagonist observed changes in how he saw his own narrative—not as a singular story of betrayal but as part of a larger tapestry that included resilience, recovery, and the strength of community. This reframe was essential to his peace of mind. He began to write, speaking publicly when he was ready, transforming his experience from isolated suffering into a force for awareness and solidarity. Sharing his story outside the therapy room was daunting but ultimately empowering, reinforcing the improvements made internally and fueling further growth.

The journey toward positive change was marked by the delicate balance between acceptance of past wounds and the courage to envision a future unchained from trauma. Medical interventions provided a crucial foundation, helping to stabilize the chaotic inner world and equip the protagonist with the means to engage fully in therapeutic healing. The side effects, while troublesome, paled in comparison to the relief found in fewer nightmares, calmer days, and a clearer mind. As he embraced these changes, his daily functioning improved in ways that touched every aspect of his life—from the intimacy of self-care to the broader scope of societal engagement.

Each step forward was a testament to both the tenacity of the human spirit and the power of compassionate care. The protagonist, once a prisoner of his trauma, began to feel the stirrings of freedom— not an immediate or total release but the fragile, precious promise of a life rebuilt, one day at a time. With every morning that brought less fear and more possibility, the positive changes solidified, laying the groundwork for an enduring recovery and a future defined not by what had been lost but by all that could be reclaimed and renewed.

Chapter 9
Rebuilding Trust

Family Reconciliation

It had been years since the tentative threads that once tied him to his family frayed completely, stretched thin by silence, shame, and the gaps wrought by his sudden departure and the slow, relentless erosion of hope. As he began to grasp the fragile outlines of healing within the sterile walls of the VA clinic, a complicated yearning started to form deep inside—a yearning to mend, to touch the fractured mosaic of his past, to reclaim a sense of belonging that had been buried beneath layers of trauma and isolation. The silence that had once been a shield now felt like a weight pressing down upon him, drawing his thoughts inexorably toward the place he had fled—a neighborhood tangled in the ghosts of his youth, where faces once familiar had transformed into shadows of suspicion, grief, and quiet reproach.

The first tentative step toward family reconciliation was not a grand gesture but a whispered promise spoken to himself in the quiet solitude of his small apartment. It was a promise to no longer remain invisible to those who had, in many ways, constituted the initial pillars of his existence, even if those pillars had been cracked and neglected under the weight of poverty, systemic oppression, and the unspoken traumas that everyone carried in their own way. Calling his mother was a moment swollen with fear and hope, a stuttering breath held for so long it seemed it might never be released. Her voice, when it came through the crackling line, was a mixture of surprise, cautious warmth, and an undercurrent of pain that years apart had deepened but never quite extinguished.

She spoke carefully at first, her words wrapped in layers of concern that barely masked a deeper uncertainty—had he truly changed? Was this the same boy who had left home with dreams of escape, who had run from the violence and squalor of the streets, only to fall into new and darker traps? But beneath the tentative questions, there was a raw, unfiltered hunger to understand, to bridge the chasm not just of miles but of experiences that had marked each of their lives in unequal measure. Conversations began slowly, scattered with pauses that felt like the reverberations of old pains, tentative threads weaving a fragile tapestry of connection. He listened as his mother spoke of the neighborhood, of relatives long gone, of the little victories and persistent struggles that had defined their collective reality while he had been away.

Meeting his father was a different challenge altogether. The memories of harsh words, missed birthdays, and the bitter legacy of generational wounds made the prospect of reunion almost unbearable. With each hesitant step toward his childhood home, the weight of years clawed at him, threatening to suffocate the fragile hope blossoming within. His father's eyes, narrowing initially in guarded recognition, hinted at the accumulated disappointment and pain that silence had long concealed. Yet beneath the scowl, there was a flicker of something older—perhaps a muted pride, a wish for redemption, or simply the human longing for connection. The conversations between them were jagged and uneven, filled with raw admissions and stumbles. They talked not only about the past but about the present struggles and the uncertain future, laying bare the complexities of a relationship battered by absence but not entirely broken.

Reconnecting with siblings was a bittersweet symphony of hesitations and tentative embraces. His younger brother, who had taken on roles he never expected, sometimes responded with resentment, as if the scars left by his absence still burned beneath the surface. Yet in moments of shared laughter, shared memories, and smoothed misunderstandings, they found fragments of unity, the subtle but profound reminder that blood ties—though tested—still held their own kind of healing alchemy. His sister's empathy was tempered by the strength born of witnessing their family's struggles firsthand, her fierce protectiveness a shield and a balm. The process of rebuilding was neither quick nor linear; it required patience, forgiveness, and the courage to confront the unspoken wounds that each of them carried.

Friends who had remained in the neighborhood occupied a unique and challenging space in his journey toward reconciliation. Some had drifted away, caught in the gravitational pull of old rhythms and patterns he had desperately tried to escape; others had held onto memories of the boy he once was, offering cautious welcome tempered by the scars of shared hardship. Reconnecting with these figures required navigating a landscape littered with old betrayals, unhealed conflicts, and the harsh realities that had shaped them all. Moments of laughter and familiarity often gave way to painful reminders of the distance he had tried to create between his past and present, underscoring the delicate balance between reintegration and self-preservation.

Beneath all these external relationships lay the perhaps greatest reconciliation of all—the painstaking journey toward mending himself. Trauma, like an invisible wound festering beneath the surface, had long distorted his sense of identity and self-worth. The years that followed the assault were marked by cycles of self-loathing and attempts at annihilation through addiction and reckless abandon. But with the gentle guidance of his therapist and the slow accumulation of small victories, he began to nurture a fragile sense of self-compassion. The process was gritty and unglamorous, marked by moments of despair, breakthroughs, and endless questioning. He grappled with the internalized shame, the fragmented memories, and the ghostly presence of his assailants, striving to reclaim agency over his own narrative.

Writing letters to family members—some sent, some tucked away in drawers—became an evocative form of self-expression, a rehearsal for verbal articulation and a tender gesture of reaching out. Each word was a relinquishment of silence, a challenge to the taboos that had shackled them all. Through these letters, he confessed not only his pain but also his hope, his fears, and his desire to rebuild a fabric torn by circumstances beyond any single person's control. Some letters received cautious replies, others no response at all, yet even the act of reaching across the divide held reverberations of change.

Family healing was complicated by the shared legacies of systemic neglect and racism that had shaped their lives long before his enlistment. Conversations often plunged into painful territory, exposing the intersections of personal trauma and collective history. It was impossible to extricate individual suffering from the broader social context—gang violence, the crack epidemic, economic deprivation, and entrenched prejudice had all left their marks in familiar and devastating patterns. In confronting these realities together, they began to perceive the roots of their mutual pain, planting the seeds for greater understanding and solidarity. The process of reconciliation thus became not only a personal endeavor but an act of communal survival, a resistance against the forces that had long sought to fracture and silence them.

Forgiveness—both given and sought—emerged as a complex terrain. It was not a linear path, nor a simplistic absolution of pain inflicted, but a multifaceted recognition of shared humanity and fractured histories. There were moments of bitter confrontation, where anger erupted in sudden storms, testing the tenuous threads of connection. There were also quiet evenings, where presence alone spoke louder than any words, offering solace in the midst of unresolved tensions. Through this interplay of conflict and compassion, the protagonist began to appreciate that reconciliation did not require forgetting or excusing but rather embracing the messy complexity of their intertwined lives.

The physicality of reunion—the awkward hugs, the tentative touches, the shared meals—served as powerful counterpoints to the emotional distance that had endured for so long. Reclaiming spaces once haunted by pain and absence felt simultaneously nostalgic and transformative. Revisiting the crumbling front porch where childhood jokes were once exchanged, sitting around a chipped kitchen table stained with years of shared history, or walking familiar streets under the dim glow of street lamps—all became rituals of reclamation. These moments embodied the fragile yet resilient heartbeat of a family striving to redefine itself amid the ruins of its past.

His family's responses to his newfound advocacy and willingness to share his story were mixed, reflecting the broader ambivalence toward confronting painful truths within the community. Some feared the stigma and potential fallout from exposing military sexual trauma; others saw his courage as a beacon illuminating dark corners previously left untouched. This delicate dynamic underscored the ongoing negotiation between personal healing and communal protection, highlighting the tensions inherent in breaking silence within closely-knit, often marginalized, families. Yet even amid hesitation, cracks of acceptance and pride began to emerge, further encouraging his journey forward.

Reconciliation also resurrected the ghosts of lost relatives—those who had passed during his absence or had been casualties of the very cycles he had once sought to escape. Their memories complicated the path with grief and remorse but also provided a spiritual tether, a reminder that healing was a continuum transcending individual lifetimes. Family stories, passed down in fragmented whispers, became threads to weave a more coherent narrative, situating his struggles in the lineage of resilience and survival.

Importantly, reconnecting with family allowed him to reimagine his own identity beyond the victimhood imposed by trauma. Through shared histories and honest dialogues, he began to reconstruct a sense of self rooted not only in pain but also in strength, heritage, and love. The act of reconciliation was, in essence, a declaration of agency—an assertion that his narrative would not be defined solely by the violence inflicted upon him but also by the bonds he chose to nurture and the future he dared to envision.

This journey was neither neat nor finished, fraught with setbacks and moments of profound vulnerability. Yet with every call answered, every visit made, and every painful conversation undertaken, the protagonist chipped away at the walls of isolation, building bridges that connected fractured hearts. Family reconciliation, once a distant hope, gradually transformed into a lived reality—one that embraced imperfection, acknowledged shared wounds, and celebrated the enduring human capacity to heal together.

New Friendships

In the fragile aftermath of trauma, when the world seems to have tilted irreversibly, the protagonist found himself cautiously navigating the treacherous landscape of relationships—those connectors to the past, anchors in the present, and bridges to the future. The assault had not only shattered his trust in others but also his faith in himself, making the prospect of reconnecting with family, friends, and even his own reflection feel like approaching a battlefield unarmed and vulnerable. Yet, there beneath the rubble of his battered self-esteem, something persistent glimmered: a yearning for connection, for understanding, for the restorative warmth of a genuine human bond.

At first, the protagonist's attempts to reestablish ties with his family were shadowed by silence and distance. His trauma was a weight none in his lineage were prepared to carry; it lingered like an invisible fog between them, suffocating the tentative embraces and wary conversations. The cultural fabric of his African American upbringing did not easily accommodate discussions of sexual assault or mental fragility—topics often cloaked in stigmatized silence or misplaced shame. Yet, slowly and unbeknownst to them all, the protagonist began to express himself through small, almost imperceptible shifts: a phone call not hung up hastily, a visit returning unfinished, a glimpse of vulnerability in moments where iron resolve had long reigned. These nascent acts, though humble in scale, became the first stitches in mending the frayed cords with his mother, siblings, and extended family, opening fissures through which empathy could seep. His mother, in particular, emerged as a silent pillar, her love a steady undercurrent despite the initial gulf of misunderstanding. She may not have always spoken the right words, but her presence—steady, unshaken—offered a silent testament to kinship that slowly began to anchor his battered spirit.

The protagonist's friendships, too, became a crucible of trial and rediscovery. Before enlisting, his social circle was a complex mosaic shaded by the harsh realities of his neighborhood: gangs, poverty, and the scars of systemic racism had shaped their lives, converse, and survival strategies. Once entrenched within the military system and later adrift in the wreckage of his trauma, many of those former friendships had frayed, severed by his absence, changed circumstances, and the invisible scars he bore. Yet, when he tentatively reached out to some of these friends, there was a mixture of surprise, relief, and caution mirrored in their responses. Some had hardened by their own ordeals; others were hesitant, unsure of how to approach the changed man before them. However, in the deliberate sharing of his pain and fears, a raw honesty began to permeate once-cautious interactions. Through late-night conversations filled with awkward silences and tentative questions, the protagonist and a handful of trusted comrades began to rebuild a fragile but authentic camaraderie, one no longer reliant on bravado or shared battles of street or military life, but on mutual recognition of vulnerability and resilience. These friendships did not erase his pain, but they offered a lifeline—a shared space where he could vent anger, admit fragility, and, crucially, understand that he was not alone in the entanglement of struggle and survival.

Perhaps the most challenging reconnection was with himself. The trauma of assault, compounded by years of addiction and homelessness, had left his identity fractured, a distorted mirror reflecting unworthiness and fear. But through the slow, difficult practice of self-compassion taught by his VA therapist, the protagonist began the painstaking process of meeting his own gaze anew. This act was an audacious reclaiming—from the deep wells of shame and silence, he learned to acknowledge his pain without capitulating to it; to recognize his worth without erasing his scars. Self-care was no longer an abstract ideal but a series of deliberate acts: rising before dawn to breathe quietly, journaling the tempestuous storms within, allowing moments of rest without guilt. Each step was a reclamation of agency, a gentle severing from the chains of self-loathing and silence that trauma had forged. The process was neither linear nor unbroken. There were days when the old voices—those insidious whispers of humiliation, fear, and despair—returned with brutal clarity. Yet, each time, the protagonist met them with a growing reservoir of resilience, bolstered by the relationships—family, friends, therapist—that stood as sentinels against his darkest moments.

Integral to this journey was his expanding exposure to new social circles, especially those within survivor support groups and VA programs. These new friendships were different, differentiated not by shared geographic roots or childhood memories, but by shared experiences of pain, survival, and the quest for healing. In these spaces, the protagonist encountered others who bore the indelible marks of MST, many of whom carried similar racial wounds. There was an unspoken language in their conversations—a rhythm of recognition and mutual validation that transcended words. With these peers, he discovered a sanctuary where judgment was absent, replaced by compassion and understanding. The collective stories woven in these rooms became tapestries of resilience, inspiring him to reimagine a future not defined by his trauma but by his capacity to rise above it. These friendships fostered a sense of belonging untainted by fear or suspicion, a balm to the isolation that trauma had incessantly fed.

Beyond the direct support groups, the protagonist's journey included connecting with individuals who challenged his perceptions in subtle yet profound ways—advocates fighting for military reform, therapists pioneering trauma-informed care, and everyday veterans whose lives were marked by complexities yet unified by dignity. These encounters broadened his horizons and infused his struggle with purpose beyond survival. He began to see himself not merely as a victim but as a potential agent of change, empowered by the network of relationships that embraced both his pain and promise.

In the quiet, unguarded moments of these relationships, whether a tentative hug, a shared laugh, or simply being held in attentive silence, the protagonist gradually knitted together something resembling wholeness. The rebuilding of trust—most crucially, trust in others and trust in himself—was a slow, nonlinear process marked by setbacks and breakthroughs. Each new friendship was both a challenge and a sanctuary, a place to test the fragile hope that perhaps connection, even after profound betrayal, was still possible.

Throughout this rebuilding, the protagonist's reflections became more nuanced. He understood now that healing was not a solitary act of will but a communal process, dependent on kindness extended and received; on the messy, imperfect work of reconciliation with those he loved and those he was learning to love within himself. The bonds formed were infused with empathy born from experience—an empathy that transcended race, rank, and circumstance to touch the raw core of human vulnerability.

Ultimately, these new friendships became the lifeblood coursing through his healing journey. They illuminated the path from desolation toward hope, from silence toward voice, from victimhood toward advocacy. They reminded him, in their varied and intricate ways, that even in the face of betrayal steeped in hate, the human heart could forge connections resilient enough to nurture recovery, affirm identity, and ignite purpose. Through the intertwined webs of family, friends, and newfound allies, the protagonist began to weave a narrative of survival marked not only by pain but by the transforming power of compassion and solidarity.

Self-Trust

Rebuilding the fragile fragments of self-trust felt like trying to piece together a shattered mirror, each shard reflecting not only the broken image of who I'd been but also the fractured distortions wrought by trauma. It was an arduous process that began not with a grand revelation or immediate breakthrough but with the quiet, almost imperceptible acts of reaching out—reaching inward and outward— towards any thread of connection remaining in a life that, for so long, had seemed irreparably tattered. The nights were still long and haunted by echoes, the silence of empty rooms pressing against me with its cold, insidious weight, but my days began to take tentative shapes around gestures of hope born from vulnerability.

It started with small conversations, the ones most would consider trivial, but, in my world, had become monumental climbs. I found myself dialing the phone, fumbling over the right words to explain I wasn't the boy who'd vanished into a nightmare, that I was still here beneath the wreckage, trying to be more than the sum of pain and fear. My mother's voice—sharp with a mixture of concern and fatigue, but unmistakably her—welcomed me hesitantly, as if unsure whether I would be another ghost or the son she remembered. The words I spoke broke through years of silence, remorse threaded beneath them like a subdued melody. "I'm trying. I want to come home. I want to fix what I broke."

It was not forgiveness I sought immediately—how could I expect that?—but rather a semblance of understanding, a beginning point where the chasms carved by betrayal might someday bridge across the abyss of silence. Slowly, she unravelled her cautious armor, sharing her pain too, her own silent battles with helplessness, hope, and the relentless worry that had shadowed every step of my absence. Our conversations were awkward and raw, often faltering in spots where unspoken grief draped heavily between us. But in the echoes of those exchanges, something vital stirred—recognition that beneath the maelstrom of my trauma, the thread of familial love remained resilient, fragile but not broken.

Friends from my past, those who weren't pushed away or lost in the spiral of my addiction and isolation, became unlikely lifelines. Rebuilding those connections demanded that I confront the shame I had buried so deeply that I had admitted not just to what had happened but to who I had become in its aftermath. It was terrifying to reveal my vulnerabilities to others, especially in a culture where strength was often measured in silence and self-reliance. Yet, their responses, when genuine, shattered some of the internalized stigma that told me I was unworthy of compassion. One friend said simply, "I'm here." Those three words, stripped of judgment and laden with quiet support, became anchors in the turbulent sea of my recovery.

But more than external relationships, the most daunting reconciliation was with myself. For years, I had waged a covert war inside, battling the voices that screamed I was weak, broken, and deserving of every ill fate that befell me. Self-trust had dissipated like mist in the harsh light of betrayal. I questioned every impulse, every decision, as if the trauma had implanted a virus of doubt in my very DNA. Could I trust my judgment, my perceptions, my emotions? Or was I forever condemned to live under the shadow of that assault, defined solely by that moment of violence?

The therapy room became a sanctuary where these questions could surface without condemnation. My therapist's patient guidance allowed me to explore the internal narratives that had governed my self-perception. Cognitive Processing Therapy (CPT) challenged me to dissect the lies I'd accepted: that I was responsible, that the world was irreparably unsafe, that my identity was forever tainted by the violation. Each session was a confrontation with the ghosts of despair and self-loathing, yet it also became a workshop for reclaiming agency. I learned that trust, especially self-trust, was less a switch to be flipped and more a muscle to be exercised gently and persistently. It was about learning to listen to my feelings without judgment, to honor the boundaries I needed, and to acknowledge the courage it took to endure and heal.

In my solitary moments, I began practicing small acts of kindness toward myself—allowing moments to pause without harsh criticism when tears came unbidden, recognizing and affirming the progress I made, no matter how incremental. I found solace in journaling, where the written word gave shape to the chaos inside me. Writing became a form of dialogue with my fragmented self, a way to articulate hopes, fears, and the faint stirrings of confidence. It was in these pages that I traced the outlines of a future where I could be whole again—not defined by trauma but in conversation with it.

Reconnecting with my body proved equally essential in reclaiming self-respect. For so long, my body had been a site of pain, a battleground where trust was violently violated. Relearning to inhabit it with grace and dignity was painfully slow. Physical activity, initially grueling and filled with resistance, transformed over time from an act of self-punishment into one of liberation. Running, stretching, even simply feeling the sun on my skin, invoked a sense of ownership I once feared lost. This bodily reclamation was intertwined with setting boundaries, learning to say no without guilt, and creating spaces—physical and emotional—where I could feel safe.

The process extended beyond the personal into my spiritual and cultural identity. Returning to the rituals and beliefs that had sustained my family through generations of hardship rekindled a sense of belonging and pride. I remembered the strength of ancestors who had faced oppression and violence, carried those scars, and yet still found ways to flourish. This connection infused my journey with a purpose bigger than my pain—a declaration that, despite the horrors inflicted upon me, I was part of an enduring legacy worthy of honor and self-love.

Yet, regaining self-trust was not linear. There were setbacks laced with overwhelming despair and days when the weight of memories threatened to suffocate any hint of confidence. Moments where doubt crept back insidiously, and I was thrust into old cycles of shame and withdrawal. But the difference lay in the growing awareness that while trauma would always be a chapter in my story, it need not be its entirety. I learned to ride the waves of emotion with grace, to surrender to vulnerability without capitulation, and to seek help without shame.

On the practical front, rebuilding trust meant I had to demonstrate to myself that I could rely on my commitments—to therapy appointments, to self-care routines, and to rebuilding relationships. Each kept promise, no matter how small, was a brick in the foundation of a renewed self-confidence. The victories, sometimes barely perceptible, accumulated into a fortress of resilience that fortified me against the corrosive effects of isolation and despair.

Family meetings, once fraught with tension and unspoken suspicions, evolved into forums of mutual support. Slowly, my relatives began to see past the scars and whispered rumors to the person striving beneath. Their acceptance and willingness to listen without judgment rekindled my faith in human connection and my own worthiness of love. In acknowledging my pain and sharing my truths, I reclaimed my narrative from the corrosive grip of silence and shame.

Among my friends, I discovered allies who not only offered companionship but also challenged the narratives that tried to knot me in self-doubt. Their unwavering presence in my storms fortified my belief that I was more than my trauma. They bore witness to my healing, celebrating milestones that once seemed unreachable and reminding me that trust, both in others and oneself, is a living, breathing endeavor.

In the quiet spaces between therapy sessions, conversations, and moments of solitude, I began to forgive myself—not in the sense of absolving guilt for acts beyond my control, but in granting myself permission to feel, to heal, and to be imperfect. Self-respect blossomed from this fertile ground of self-compassion, grounding me in a reality where my worth was intrinsic, not predicated on the cruel acts inflicted upon me.

This blossoming self-trust reshaped my future outlook. Where once I saw only the abyss of pain and hopelessness, I started to perceive possibilities—relationships rebuilt, a vocation reclaimed, a life redesigned with intention rather than survival instinct alone. It fueled my advocacy, giving voice to those silenced by fear and stigma, and stoked a resolve to transform personal tragedy into societal change.

Though scars would remain—etched deep in mind and body—they no longer dictated the contours of my existence. I had learned that to trust oneself after betrayal is a brave act of rebellion against despair. It is a slow dance of courage, persistence, and grace, one that I continue to navigate every day with a spirit increasingly defined by hope rather than fear. In this reclaimed self-trust, I found the seed from which healing grows, and from which life, once again, blossoms.

Chapter 10
Speaking Out

Overcoming Fear

Fear clung to him like a shadow, relentless and suffocating. It was a constant companion in the days, weeks, and months that followed the unspeakable betrayal he endured. Fear that his story would be met with disbelief or dismissal. Fear that those he trusted would turn their backs, judging him instead of supporting. Fear that speaking his truth would unravel whatever fragile sense of dignity he had left, dragging him into further isolation. The very idea of opening up about what happened felt like exposing every vulnerability he had spent years trying to bury beneath layers of silence and pain. Yet, beneath the crushing weight of anxiety, there was a flicker of something unexpected—a cautious, trembling hope that maybe, by telling his story, he could reclaim the power that was stolen from him.

It took a heavy toll to even contemplate breaking the silence. For years, the entrenched military culture he had entered preached loyalty, toughness, and self-reliance, all of which seemed incompatible with expressions of vulnerability. Admitting to being a victim of something as stigmatized and misunderstood as Military Sexual Trauma threatened not only his reputation but his very sense of identity. He was supposed to be strong, to bear the burdens without complaint, to embody resilience. Yet, the assault shattered that illusion, leaving an aching gap between who he was expected to be and the shattered pieces of who he had become. The societal expectations around manhood, particularly within the framework of his African American community and the military institution, compounded the shame. To the outside world, confessing such an ordeal was akin to confessing a weakness so profound that it could ostracize him from both worlds.

The anxiety of potential backlash was not unfounded. He had witnessed firsthand how survivors, especially men of color, were often met with skepticism or outright hostility. The fear of retaliation—whether covert or overt—loomed large. Threats hung in his memory like specters, originating not just from the perpetrators but from a system that seemed designed to silence and deter him. The military's hierarchical structure and rigid code of silence created an environment where breaking ranks could mean alienation, harassment, or worse. He knew that some in command might prefer the problem to disappear quietly rather than face the inconvenient truth of racial hatred intertwining with sexual violence within their ranks. His family's safety was another layer of fear that complicated his decision to come forward. The threats against them echoed in his mind; he worried that confessing his trauma could inadvertently endanger those he loved most.

Yet, amidst the daunting fear, there was a profound and growing realization that silence was a far more dangerous prison. Every day he refrained from sharing his experience was a day the trauma tightened its grip, informing his nightmares, poisoning his self-worth, and chaining him to the past. The internalized shame whispered that he was tainted, that his worth was diminished, that he had failed somehow. But as he engaged in therapy, guided by a compassionate VA therapist who understood the intersection of race, trauma, and military culture, the narrative began to shift. He learned that his truth was not a mark of weakness but a testament to his bravery. The very act of contemplating telling his story was in itself an act of courage and defiance against the forces that sought to silence him.

This transformation did not happen overnight. Each small step out of the shadows felt like wading through a storm without an umbrella. He practiced telling parts of his story quietly, tentatively, sometimes just vowing to himself that one day he would say it out loud. The therapist provided a sanctuary where judgment was absent, and empathy was abundant. Here, he found the language to articulate his pain, to decode the tangled web of emotions left by the assault—shame, anger, confusion, grief. Cognitive Processing Therapy helped him reframe the story he had told himself about what happened, challenging the irrational beliefs that held him captive. It was during these sessions that he began to confront the core of his fear: the idea that he was alone, that nobody would believe him, that his life would be irreparably damaged by breaking silence.

Armed with new understanding and a fragile but growing sense of self-compassion, he gradually allowed himself to reach out beyond the therapist's office. Sharing his experience with trusted comrades and a close friend became a turning point. Though heart-pounding and vulnerable, their responses were unexpectedly supportive, helping to erode years of self-doubt. These encounters illuminated how much stigma was tied to ignorance—a cruel misconception that survivors were somehow complicit or responsible for the violence inflicted upon them. By speaking, he was not only challenging that misconception but also connecting with others who had suffered in silence, discovering that he was far from isolated.

The ripple effects were profound. Every time he spoke, no matter how painful, the invisible weight on his chest lightened slightly. The story of betrayal no longer belonged solely to him but became a bridge to collective awareness, a beacon for other survivors who might be wrestling with similar fears. His voice, once muffled by dread, grew stronger and clearer. Yet, with each public breath he took, he was acutely aware of the possibility of backlash—judgment from those who couldn't understand, rejection from the very institution that failed to protect him, and the impersonal machinery of bureaucracy that reduced his trauma to statistics and paperwork. But the alternative—perpetual silence, invisibility, and despair—felt far worse.

Facing potential backlash and shame demanded more than sheer willpower; it required reclaiming his narrative on his terms. He recognized that telling his story was not about re-traumatizing himself but about transforming trauma into testimony—one that could illuminate systemic failures and humanize the statistics too often cloaked in euphemisms. By breaking the chains of silence, he opened a door not only for his healing but also for institutional accountability. In public forums, support groups, and conversations with policymakers, his courage sparked dialogues that had been long overdue. Suddenly, the assault was no longer an anomaly tucked away in the shadows but a painful reality demanding urgent attention and reform.

This bold vulnerability was, paradoxically, an act of empowerment. He wielded truth as a weapon against stigma, dismantling the narratives that marginalized survivors and silenced their pain. The shame that had once seemed insurmountable began eroding, replaced by a quiet pride—not in the assault itself, but in the resilience that survival had cultivated. He was no longer just the victim of a horrific act but a survivor who chose to redefine what strength meant in the face of profound trauma. This redefinition extended beyond himself, offering hope to others chained by fear, demonstrating that courage was not the absence of fear but the determination to move forward despite it.

His story, once buried beneath years of silence, became a testament to the complex interplay of racial violence, systemic betrayal, and personal resilience. In shedding light on these intersecting horrors, he challenged the military institution to confront uncomfortable truths and to strive for genuine transformation in how it supports survivors, especially those from marginalized communities. His courage was an invitation to society at large to listen, to empathize, and most importantly, to act.

As he stood on the precipice of sharing his story more widely, memories of threats and the specter of shame lingered faintly at the edges of his consciousness. But they no longer defined him. Instead, he held onto the knowledge that his voice was a vital thread in the tapestry of change—one that could weave understanding, foster healing, and dismantle the silence that had long perpetuated pain. Overcoming fear was not a singular moment of triumph but an ongoing journey marked by commitment, bravery, and the unwavering belief that telling the truth was a path toward reclaiming life and dignity. Each word spoken was a step forward, an affirmation that despite the betrayal he endured, he would not be broken, muted, or forgotten. Instead, his story would echo beyond himself, inspiring others to find their voices and confront the darkness that had too long gone unchallenged.

Finding a Voice

For the longest time, the weight of silence pressed heavily on him, a crushing burden that seemed inseparable from his very soul. The trauma he had endured was a secret, locked deep inside, fenced off by layers of shame, fear, and the haunting threat that had been impressed upon him from the moment his world shattered—any attempt to speak out would invite retaliation, harm to those he loved, and the final erasure of his dignity. Yet, amid that suffocating silence, a flicker of something stubborn and persistent began to grow. It was the tiniest spark of courage, a quiet but unyielding urge that whispered insistently: "You deserve to be heard. Your story matters." Finding a voice was not an overnight transformation; it was a painstaking, deliberate process that demanded dismantling the walls he had built for self-protection and stepping, trembling and uncertain, into the blinding light of truth.

The courage to confront stigma, especially when it stemmed from the very institution he had once believed would shield him, was colossal. For years, he had carried the invisible scars inflicted not only by the violent assault itself but by the systemic failure that perpetuated denial and silence. The military, a place where loyalty and brotherhood were idolized, had been twisted into a crucible of betrayal. Each step toward telling his truth felt like unraveling a complex web of compounded fears: the fear of being labeled weak or broken, the fear of disbelief or dismissal, the fear of being further ostracized as a Black man in a predominantly white, hierarchical system that had tacitly allowed such heinous acts to persist. These fears were not unfounded. Military culture had long prized silence on matters deemed shameful, and victims of sexual assault often found themselves pushed into margins where their pain was minimized or outright ignored. Breaking this silence meant risking not only personal safety but also the fragile social connections he had left, the tenuous bonds of trust he struggled to rebuild.

Yet, the act of sharing began as a delicate, almost clandestine exercise. In the early stages, it was expressed in guarded conversations with a select few—friends he trusted not because they gave easy solace, but because they held space for his pain without judgment. These moments, though fleeting and vulnerable, became the scaffolding that supported his burgeoning voice. He realized that speaking was not a one-time act; it was an ongoing negotiation with his own pain and the reactions of listeners who often grappled with discomfort or disbelief. Over time, as he engaged with survivor networks and therapists, he encountered others whose stories resonated with his own, and this shared experience became a powerful catalyst. It revealed that the trauma was widespread, that he was not alone and not to blame, and that by speaking, he could transform personal agony into collective strength. This community of voices was a radical counterpoint to the imposed silence, a chorus that refused to be stifled.

One of the most profound challenges was dismantling the internalized stigma that had taken residence within him long before external judgment could. The assault left deep wounds of self-doubt and self-condemnation; he wrestled endlessly with thoughts that questioned his worth and right to healing. Every time he considered coming forward, a silent, relentless voice echoed that he was damaged beyond repair, that revealing the truth would only contribute to his shame and cancel whatever agency he still possessed. But gradually, through therapy and the relentless encouragement of his therapist, he learned that courage did not mean the absence of fear but the decision to move forward despite it. He discovered that vulnerability was not weakness but a form of profound strength—an act of reclaiming power from those who had sought to strip it away. There was an alchemical transformation in this process: pain transmuted into purpose, trauma's chaos channelled into narrative coherence. He began to write—first in journals, then in letters, and ultimately in testimonies shared with advocacy groups and public forums. Writing became a sanctuary, a projective space where he could order his fragmented experiences into coherent, comprehensible stories.

The impact of telling his truth rippled far beyond his own healing journey, seeping into the lives of others who had long lived in quiet suffering. Each public disclosure—whether in community meetings, survivor panels, or online platforms—was met with a surge of mixed emotions: fear of backlash, relief in catharsis, and a tentative exhilaration born from speaking boldly against entrenched silence. Many survivors reached out, telling him their own stories with gratitude and a sense of solidarity. For the first time, his narrative became a source of empowerment not only for himself but for a network of individuals marginalized by trauma and institutional neglect. He witnessed how his words could challenge entrenched myths about MST and reshape the conversation, humanizing survivors in a way statistics and official reports could not. This shared vulnerability began to chip away at the stigma that surrounded MST, confronting the cultural and institutional indifference so often weaponized against victims. His advocacy work took shape not from a sense of obligation but from a deep, visceral understanding that change was possible—and that silence was not an option.

Publicly revealing his assault also brought fresh waves of pain and resistance. Not all reactions were supportive; some dismissed or questioned his motives, others deployed coded racisms or cast doubts on his credibility. There were moments when the wrath of denial felt like a second assault: a constant reminder that societal and military structures still failed to protect or even acknowledge victims. Yet each challenge reaffirmed the necessity of his voice in the conversation. He resolved that if his truth could unsettle the comfortable denials of power, if it could provoke discomfort that led to reflection and eventually reform, then every ounce of suffering endured in exposure was an investment in a better future for those who would come after. He learned to navigate this contentious space with grace and resolve, leaning on allies within MST advocacy groups, mental health professionals, and fellow survivors who fortified his resilience.

The therapeutic process had prepared him to articulate not only his story but also the complex emotions that accompanied it. He was no longer merely a victim recounting events but a thoughtful agent of change, articulating the intersections of race, institutional abuse, and systemic negligence. He understood that his voice carried a rare and necessary perspective in a dialogue often dominated by sanitized narratives or statistical abstractions. His testimony illuminated the racial violence embedded within the military's landscape, exposing how hate groups like the KKK permeated the ranks with impunity, exerting terror not only physically but psychologically. By embracing this uncomfortable truth, he disrupted the myth of the military as a uniform sanctuary and underscored the urgent need for comprehensive reform.

Over time, his story took on multiple forms and found diverse audiences. He spoke in small support groups, where his words provided solace and validation to others dragging similar ghosts. He contributed essays to survivor-focused publications, translating personal pain into collective awareness. He was invited to panels with government officials and policymakers, where his firsthand experience catalyzed discussions about systemic changes to reporting, prevention, and care services within the military and Veteran Affairs. Each setting demanded a different modulation of his narrative, balancing candor with strategic emphasis on advocacy goals. This adaptability underscored the evolving nature of finding a voice—it was not a fixed, singular act but a dynamic process of listening, refining, and reaching out.

Perhaps the most poignant and symbolic moment of reclaiming his voice came when he stood before a crowd of veterans and military personnel at a conference dedicated to MST awareness. The room, filled with hundreds who could relate to varying degrees of his pain, was thick with emotion. Speaking aloud, in that charged space, he felt the paradox of vulnerability and strength converge. His words were raw and unfiltered, capturing not only the horror but also the resilience sewn through his journey. Tears traced paths down cheeks—his own and those in the audience—as walls of isolation cracked wide open. It was not an easy speech; some moments faltered. Yet it marked a powerful breakthrough—the transformation from silenced victim to vocal survivor, from invisible suffering to unignorable reality.

Through telling his story, he also confronted his own fractured identity. The assault had not only compromised his physical and mental safety but had fractured his sense of self. It had inserted a dangerous narrative about powerlessness that he struggled to untangle for years. But by speaking the truth aloud, he confronted those lies head-on. He began to see himself not merely in the shadow of victimhood but as a whole person, complex and multifaceted—capable of love, healing, and purpose. His voice became a bridge between the person he was before the assault and the person he was becoming. It allowed him to reclaim autonomy, rewrite the narrative, and chart a path forward defined not by trauma but by hope and strength.

Ultimately, finding a voice was an act of profound radical self-respect and defiance. It demanded he stare into the abyss of his darkest moments and say, "I will not be erased." It meant breaking through the insulated silence of institutional indifference and societal denial, holding up his truth as both testimony and testament. And it required immense trust—in himself, in others, and in the possibility that sharing his pain might ignite transformation. His journey from silence to speech was neither neat nor linear. It was jagged and painful but deeply human and necessary. By choosing to tell his story, he offered himself—and through himself, countless others—the chance to be seen, heard, and ultimately, to heal.

Community Response

The moment the story unfolded beyond the intimate walls of therapy sessions and private confessions, it carried a weight that extended far past the protagonist's singular ordeal. His decision to lay bare the darkest corners of his military experience—the raw, unfiltered truth of his assault and the deep, corrosive wounds it inflicted—was an act that demanded immense courage. It was an act that challenged the rigid silence that had long cloaked Military Sexual Trauma in shadows, an act that defied the stigmas suffocating survivors across the nation. When his story began to circulate, the response from the community—veterans, survivors, and the public alike—was complex, layered with discomfort, empathy, resistance, and ultimately, a profound respect for the bravery it embodied.

Among veterans, the reaction reflected the fractured, often complicated nature of military culture itself. The military, as an institution, is built on principles of strength, resilience, and unity, yet when confronted with something as unsettling as sexual violence perpetrated within its ranks, the response was initially fragmented. Some veterans expressed palpable surprise, shocked that such brutality could exist in a system designed to protect its own. Others were defensive, grappling with feelings of betrayal or denial, unwilling at first to confront the bleak reality that their brotherhood and sisterhood might harbor such darkness. Yet as his courage in telling his truth became apparent, many veterans found their perspectives shifting. For those who had suffered in silence—whether from trauma, discrimination, or isolation—the story served as a beacon, a signal that they were not alone. His candid narration gave voice to those unnamed, unseen wounds festering beneath uniforms and medals. It became a catalyst for veterans to come forward, to share their own experiences, and to seek solidarity in the shared pain and solace found within community.

Survivors of Military Sexual Trauma responded with a mixture of validation and relief, tempered with an acute awareness of the long, arduous path of recovery. Hearing his experience articulated in such honesty was more than just an acknowledgment of their struggles; it was a shattering of invisibility. The protagonist became a figure not just of victimhood, but of resilience and defiance. For many, his story rekindled memories long buried, stirring both anguish and a cautious hope. The shared experience illuminated the common threads of betrayal and silence, but also the possibilities of healing through openness and connection. The impact was particularly profound within marginalized groups—Black veterans and other minority survivors—who often bear the compounded burdens of racial trauma alongside sexual violence. His narrative validated the particular intersections of race and victimization within the military context, breaking down the isolation forced upon them by both systemic racism and stigma around sexual assault. As word spread, networks of survivors began to strengthen, rallying around the message that confronting trauma was not a sign of weakness but an act of unyielding strength.

Public reaction, meanwhile, was an endlessly evolving tapestry of acknowledgement, discomfort, and, in many quarters, awakening. Initially, many who encountered his story struggled to reconcile the stark reality of military sexual violence with their perceptions of the military as an honorable, disciplined protector of the nation. The cognitive dissonance was palpable—how could an institution so revered harbor such dangerous failures? This disjoint sparked vital conversations, both in traditional media and in grassroots spaces, about the systemic issues within military culture that allowed such assaults to go unchecked. His story became a rallying point for advocacy groups, human rights organizations, and mental health professionals, fueling campaigns aimed at reforming military policies, increasing survivor support, and demanding accountability. The ripples reached lawmakers and policymakers, stirring debates that crossed party lines and focused beyond the confines of the Pentagon.

Yet beyond the waves of response and social discourse lay the quieter, less visible shifts in attitudes—the subtle but profound ways in which individual minds and hearts began to change. For many members of the public, hearing a survivor's voice resonate so openly forced a reckoning with their own biases and assumptions. The stigma surrounding sexual assault, particularly within the hyper-masculine and regimented military sphere, often silences survivors, cloaking them in shame and disbelievers' shadows. His courage pierced through this oppressive silence, challenging stereotypes and dismantling preconceived narratives about strength, vulnerability, and identity. People began to understand that trauma does not discriminate by rank, race, or creed; it is an insidious force that requires compassion and intervention. Survivorship was reclaimed from silence and shame and reframed as a testament to human endurance.

The protagonist's confrontation with stigma, both internal and external, was a monumental feat. Internally, confronting years of self-blame, guilt, and secrecy demanded a profound reimagining of self-worth. Pronouncing his trauma aloud amid public scrutiny was a defiant rejection of the shame his assailants intended to impose. This act also shattered the pervasive myth that silence protects survivors or the institution; instead, it demonstrated that truth and transparency can be revolutionary acts of self-advocacy and healing. Externally, he faced skepticism, ignorance, and dismissal from some quarters, but also unwavering support from others who recognized the urgent need to listen without judgment. Gradually, this stubborn perseverance transformed into a bridge linking isolated survivors to a broader community committed to recognition, justice, and reform.

The impact of telling his truth reverberated beyond personal healing; it became a platform for advocacy and systemic change. Community forums, support groups, and advocacy events welcomed his testimony, lending a powerful firsthand account to otherwise abstract discussions about Military Sexual Trauma. His narrative humanized the statistics, transforming them from cold numbers into lived realities that demand attention and empathy. The courage to share his experience encouraged military leadership and policymakers to take concrete steps toward improving reporting mechanisms, protection measures, and therapeutic resources for victims. Moreover, his journey underscored the essential need for cultural shifts within military ranks—dismantling the toxic masculinity, racism, and complicity that perpetuate cycles of violence. His story became a clarion call for accountability, transparency, and reform.

For the broader survivor community, his story was a call to reclaim agency—to move beyond victimhood into advocacy, to transform silence into solidarity, and to anchor healing in shared experience. The courage to speak out illuminated the path for others, offering hope that the darkness of trauma could not, and would not, define their futures. As public awareness grew, the collective stigma began to erode, replaced with understanding that trauma responses are complex and that empathy, not judgment, is the appropriate societal response. Mental health professionals and veteran services saw a surge in outreach, reflecting a growing willingness among survivors to seek help and a recognition of the need for accessible, culturally competent care.

In the end, the community's response to his story became a testament to the power of courage in the face of overwhelming adversity. It was a reminder that healing from trauma is not a solitary journey but a communal endeavor that requires allies, advocates, and systemic transformation. His voice, once silenced by fear and trauma, grew into a chorus echoing through communities yearning for justice and compassion. It underscored that confronting stigma is perhaps the greatest act of bravery of all—the courage to stand unflinching in one's truth, to challenge entrenched silence and shame, and to illuminate the path forward for those who follow. The impact of this confrontation rippled outward, fostering empathy, igniting change, and affirming that survivors' stories, no matter how painful, are essential threads in the fabric of a just and humane society.

Chapter 11
Advocacy and Hope

Joining Forces

The hesitant first steps toward connection often feel like walking into a room filled with shadows. For someone whose silence has been their constant companion, whose trauma has been locked away behind walls thick with shame and fear, finding others who truly understand can be a beacon of fragile hope. It was these cautious, trembling strides into the world of survivor groups that began to stitch together the fraying fragments of his shattered spirit. The idea of opening up—of exposing wounds, rough and raw to others—was terrifying beyond measure at first. He had learned, painfully, that not all ears wanted to listen, not all eyes sought to see. But within the walls of survivor meetings, or through conversations stitched by phone lines and online forums, something shifted; the heavy burden he carried was no longer his alone, and in that shared pain lay the surprising tenderness of empathy and understanding.

Joining survivor groups was more than an act of seeking solace; it was a revolutionary act of reclaiming agency. These groups, often comprised of individuals from diverse backgrounds, united by the common thread of military sexual trauma, stood as living testaments to resilience. For him, attending these gatherings marked the first real opportunity to hear voices echoing experiences too similar to be coincidence and too diverse to be uniform. There were retellings of nightmares and day-to-day battles, but also stories of survival—of finding light after an abyss that seemed endless. In these collective truths, he found a mirror reflecting not just his suffering but a blueprint for healing. The presence of fellow survivors who navigated the labyrinthine systems of military and veteran affairs illuminated paths once obscured by confusion and dread.

The survivor groups became crucibles not only of personal restoration but of empowerment. Conversations flowed beyond mere venting sessions, evolving into strategic discussions about the institutional frameworks that had failed them all so profoundly. They dissected policies that perpetuated silence and invisibility, analyzed military protocols that rendered victims invisible and perpetrators empowered. In these dialogues, his personal story, once locked inside a vault of self-protection, intertwined with the broader tapestry of systemic failure and the urgent need for reform. The collective voices grew stronger, resonant with determination, issuing a quiet but unyielding call for change. For the first time, his role expanded—no longer just a victim struggling to survive, but an advocate wielding narrative and truth as instruments of transformation.

Participating in workshops and advocacy training sessions provided the tools to channel overwhelming pain into articulate action. There was an intoxicating sense of power in learning how to communicate his experience with clarity and purpose, to stand before policymakers or media representatives and demand accountability not from abstract institutions but from flesh-and-blood individuals entrusted with safeguarding those under their command. His meetings with lawmakers and military leaders were daunting arenas, yet they underscored a profound shift within him. He was not just recounting his trauma; he was contextualizing it within the lived realities of countless others, illuminating the intersections of racism, sexual violence, and institutional indifference with unwavering candor. These encounters laid bare the entrenched resistance to acknowledging and addressing MST, but simultaneously sparked a growing chorus for transparency and justice.

In these moments of advocacy, the pain that had once threatened to consume him transmuted into purpose. He spoke not only for himself but for every survivor who had been silenced by fear or disbelief. At times, the process was exhausting—rekindling memories that clawed at his composure—but the solidarity found in these rooms provided a tether to endurance. The collective force of survivors standing shoulder to shoulder was a palpable reminder that the shadows of trauma could be pierced by communal courage. Each policy meeting or public forum where he shared his story became a battleground where truth clashed with denial, but his voice was steadfast, anchored in the authenticity of lived experience.

The survivor groups also fostered invaluable friendships born of mutual respect and vulnerability. Some comrades had walked similar paths, escaping environments suffocated by violence and hatred, only to be betrayed within the very institution sworn to protect them. Their shared histories of encountering racial animus and systemic neglect deepened their bonds beyond mere camaraderie. Within these relationships, laughter occasionally blossomed amidst tears, moments of lightness carving out sacred spaces of relief. The exchange of coping strategies, referrals to therapists familiar with military sexual trauma, and guidance on navigating Veterans Affairs' often opaque processes created a support network essential for survival and renewal. The experiential wisdom embedded within these groups was sometimes the only compass available in moments of despair.

Alongside these intimate engagements, he immersed himself in broader advocacy initiatives aimed at raising public awareness about MST. Collaborations with national organizations dedicated to veterans' rights and sexual assault prevention opened channels to reach wider audiences. He contributed articles and personal essays that peeled back the veneer of military pride to reveal the human cost beneath. At public speaking events, he stood before varied crowds— military personnel, policymakers, community activists—and with every measured word, chipped away at the stigma and silence that cloaked MST. His narrative became a bridge, linking personal pain to collective consciousness, urging society to recognize and rectify the invisible wounds borne by so many. The power of storytelling in advocacy was profound; by bearing witness to his own suffering, he summoned empathy and understanding where apathy once reigned.

This involvement illuminated the inseparability of the personal and the political in the fight against MST. Survivor groups were not mere sanctuaries for healing but dynamic spaces where lived experiences catalyzed institutional scrutiny and reform. Working alongside attorneys, mental health professionals, and veterans' advocates, he engaged in drafting policy recommendations that tackled the inadequacies of military justice and victim support systems. The painstaking process of advocacy required patience and resilience in the face of bureaucratic inertia but also instilled a sense of collective agency. Having once felt powerless amid a culture of silence and intimidation, contributing to tangible policy shifts instilled a deep, albeit cautious, hope for transformation.

The journey through survivor groups also brought into sharp focus the pervasive racial undertones entwined with acts of violence and systemic neglect within the military. Conversations revealed how racial prejudice amplified vulnerability, with his own harrowing experience at the hands of white supremacists within the ranks serving as a stark exemplar. This acknowledgment within the community underscored the necessity of intersectional advocacy—where combatting MST could not be disentangled from addressing racism and hate-based violence. The articulation of these intertwined oppressions enriched the movement's complexity, challenging oversimplified narratives often presented to the public and policymakers. In this way, survivor groups functioned as vital incubators of critical dialogue that widened the scope of understanding and advocacy.

His engagement with these communities also facilitated a reclamation of identity fragmented by trauma. Through group sharing, he confronted the scars inflicted not only by assault but also by internalized shame fostered by a military culture steeped in hypermasculinity and silence around vulnerability. Witnessing others embrace their truth without apology emboldened him to dismantle his own self-recriminations. The gradual process of self-acceptance was neither linear nor painless, but the collective witness of survivor networks offered both refuge and resolve. By affirming each other's worth and dignity, these groups became sanctuaries where the oppressive weight of stigma was gradually lifted, creating space for genuine healing.

Moreover, survivor groups championed practical assistance crucial for navigating the labyrinthine systems dealing with veterans' health and justice. Guided by peers who had traversed similar bureaucratic mazes, he gained insights into securing medical care, psychological support, and legal representation. The advocacy efforts extended to ensuring that military sexual trauma was formally recognized in disability claims and benefits decisions—an essential step for numerous survivors seeking not only acknowledgment but tangible support. Connecting with these resources mitigated the pervasive isolation common among MST victims, anchoring him within a network where survival was collectively fought and shared. This ripple effect from individual narrative to systemic assistance illustrated the profound interconnectedness of personal recovery and structural accountability.

One of the most transformative outcomes of his involvement emerged in the opportunities to educate military leadership and fellow service members about MST prevention and response. Survivor groups frequently partnered with military institutions to facilitate training sessions aimed at dismantling harmful norms and cultivating cultures of respect and safety. While resistance and denial were at times palpable, the presence of survivors speaking honestly about their experiences humanized issues often buried beneath statistics and reports. The courage exhibited in these educational endeavors—the willingness to face skeptical or dismissive audiences—demonstrated the potential for change rooted in vulnerability and truth. Knowing that his testimony might prevent others from enduring similar betrayals instilled a renewed sense of purpose beyond personal healing.

His growth within survivor communities also transformed his self-perception—not merely as someone wounded by past injustices but as an agent of change bridging the chasm between silence and speech, invisibility and recognition. The gradual shift from survivor to advocate was marked by moments of fear and exhilaration as he testified before military panels, contributed to documentaries, and lobbied for legislative reforms aimed at improving accountability and resources for MST victims. These public platforms were battlegrounds for competing narratives. Still, with each appearance, he reclaimed sovereignty over his narrative, reshaping identity from that of a broken victim to a resilient, determined voice for collective justice.

Through his involvement with survivor groups, he also recognized the power of intersectionality—the understanding that his experience as a Black man subjected to racialized sexual violence demanded a nuanced approach to advocacy and healing. This awareness propelled collaborations with organizations addressing racial justice, LGBTQ+ veteran rights, and trauma-informed care, broadening the reach and depth of MST activism. Such alliances challenged militarized norms that favored homogeneity and silence, advocating instead for inclusive environments where diversity of experience and identity was not just tolerated but valued and protected. These coalitions enriched his advocacy work, making it more attuned to the realities faced by marginalized survivors and more impactful in effecting systemic change.

Being part of survivor groups was also a masterclass in resilience and hope. Witnessing peers navigate seemingly insurmountable struggles and emerge with renewed strength served as a source of inspiration. Stories of rebuilding families, pursuing education, or creating art from pain were woven into the fabric of group meetings, infusing conversations with light amid darkness. These narratives reinforced that the journey from victimhood to survivorship, though fraught and complex, was possible. The collective wisdom reminded him that healing was not a finite destination but an ongoing process shaped by community, courage, and commitment. This shared knowledge fortified him when confronting setbacks, reminding him that he was not alone and that survival was an act of defiance against the forces that sought to silence and destroy.

The connection forged within survivor groups instilled a profound sense of belonging, countering the isolation inflicted by trauma and systemic neglect. This newfound community became a vital element not only for emotional sustenance but also for practical support during crises. Whether it was accompanying a fellow survivor to a medical appointment, sharing housing resources during periods of homelessness, or simply offering a listening ear during moments of despair, the bonds crystallized into lifelines. This reciprocity reinforced the transformative power of shared experience and mutual aid, grounding his recovery in tangible expressions of care and solidarity. Through these connections, he discovered that healing was both inward and outward—anchored in personal resolve and nurtured by collective strength.

In these survivor spaces, laughter occasionally broke through the sorrow, a soundtrack of triumph woven into the narrative of pain. Shared humor—sometimes dark, sometimes absurd—acted as a balm, a reminder of the enduring humanity beneath trauma's scars. Celebrating small victories, from a successful therapy session to a new job or public speaking engagement, created communal rituals that honored resilience. These moments punctuated the arduous journey with reminders that life, though altered, still held richness and possibility. They nurtured hope, a fragile yet fierce force that propelled him forward when despair threatened to reclaim its hold.

The role of survivor groups extended beyond healing and advocacy to shaping a legacy. By mentoring newcomers, sharing resources, and participating in training future advocates, he contributed to a continuum of support that would endure long after his own story was told. His willingness to stand in the spotlight encouraged others to emerge from the shadows, cultivating a movement that transcended individual narratives to forge collective momentum. In this way, survivor groups were crucibles of transformation—places where pain was reframed as power, silence converted to speech, and isolation replaced by community. They represented both the scars and the salve of a journey marked by unspeakable betrayal but also remarkable resilience.

Ultimately, connecting with survivor groups rekindled a faith in humanity and justice that trauma had nearly extinguished. The journey was neither linear nor easy, burdened by setbacks and moments of vulnerability, but it illuminated a path forward. Through shared struggles and triumphs, the bleak landscape of betrayal gave way to a terrain marked by courage, advocacy, and hope. In joining forces with others who bore similar burdens, he found not only healing but purpose—an unyielding commitment to transform pain into progress, to ensure that no survivor would ever again face the shadows alone. The bonds forged within these groups became a lifeline, an anchor, and the foundation from which a battered but unbroken spirit could rise.

Raising Awareness

The journey toward raising awareness felt to me like stepping onto a vast, jagged frontier where shadows clung tightly to the edges of truth. For so long, the stories of survivors like me—the voiceless, the silenced, the broken—had been hidden beneath layers of shame and institutional denial. But the air grew thicker with urgency, and I knew that to break the cycle, I had to step beyond my personal healing and become a beacon for others still trapped in darkness. My first tentative steps into public speaking were uneven, trembling with vulnerability and the ever-present fear of judgment. Standing before a crowd, eyes fixed intently upon me, I grappled with the sharp sting of recalling memories I wanted buried but knew I had to unearth. Each word was a piece of flesh torn open, each sentence a raw nerve exposed. Yet, ironically, this exposure brought with it a strange sort of strength—a power born not of perfection but of authenticity. It was in these moments, recounting my painful past as a victim of military sexual trauma at the hands of those sworn to protect, that I began to wield my voice not as a weapon of self-punishment but as a tool of transformation.

The initial forums were small—local support group meetings, veteran centers, community gatherings—but they became foundational pillars upon which my advocacy was built. I learned that sharing my narrative was not just about unburdening myself; it was about lighting sparks in others hesitant to speak, about shattering the silence that too often fed the epidemic of MST. As I grew more comfortable, the invitations multiplied, reaching state-wide conferences and national forums dedicated to veterans' rights and mental health. At these events, my story became intertwined with broader dialogues on systemic injustice, racial violence, and institutional neglect. I wove my past experiences with hard facts and statistics, marshaling evidence of the staggering prevalence of MST and the disproportionate impact on Black service members. It was crucial to me that my advocacy never veer into a solitary lament but resonate as a clarion call demanding systemic accountability and reform.

Building connections with organizations focused on military sexual trauma became the next critical step. I sought out alliances with established groups like Service Women's Action Network, Protect Our Defenders, and the Military Rape Crisis Center, learning from their seasoned expertise while offering the vital perspective of an African American male survivor—an often overlooked demographic in the broader MST conversation. Together, we designed outreach initiatives that combined education with empowerment, focusing on creating safe spaces for survivors to be heard without judgment and without fear of retribution. Our collaborations raised awareness through public campaigns, survivor testimonies, workshops tailored for military personnel, and an impactful social media presence. These joint efforts sought to dismantle the toxic cultures within military ranks that allowed such violations to fester unchecked. I was no longer just a voice; I had become part of a wider chorus demanding that the military reckon with its failures.

Getting involved in policy advocacy required a new skill set. Engaging with legislators, military officials, and advocacy groups required not only passion but also patience and strategic acumen. I spent hours studying bills, learning about the intricacies of veteran affairs policies, and attending congressional hearings—often as an outside spectator before mustering the courage to speak firsthand. The challenge lay in confronting bureaucratic inertia and sometimes outright hostility. There were moments when the coldness of institutional corridors and the skepticism of some officials felt suffocating. Yet, with each meeting, I sharpened my message, emphasizing that the military's neglect of sexual assault wasn't just a moral failing but a security risk, threatening the cohesion and effectiveness of the ranks. I underscored the specific intersection of race and sexual violence, pushing for policies that recognized the unique barriers Black survivors face—including fear of retribution, lack of cultural sensitivity in support services, and compounded trauma from systemic racism.

Testifying before legislative committees marked pivotal moments in my advocacy. My voice, once burdened with silence and shame, now resonated with a stern and unwavering demand for justice. Sharing my story in those austere chambers was nerve-wracking but vital. I described the heinous assault in clinical and honest detail, refusing to dilute the horror in an effort to spare sensitivity. It was essential that lawmakers grasp the full gravity of MST and its lifelong repercussions. I spoke not only for myself but also for countless veterans whose pain remained invisible. The gravity of my testimony was matched by a growing audience of policymakers and media eager to expose military sexual trauma's prevalence and push for systemic overhaul. Some lawmakers responded with empathy and a genuine desire to effect change, offering commitments to fund better prevention programs, ensure victim confidentiality, and expand access to trauma-informed care. Others remained hesitant, constrained by political calculations or entrenched military culture, resistant to transparency.

Beyond formal hearings, grassroots outreach formed the bedrock of my advocacy. I traveled to military bases, community centers, and universities, standing alongside fellow survivors, veteran advocates, and allies to conduct workshops and panel discussions. These sessions encouraged frank conversations about consent, power dynamics, racial hostility, and the lasting impacts of MST. For many attendees, especially young recruits, these were moments of awakening—a chance to see the military not just as a path to stability but as an institution fraught with potential dangers that must be confronted. I shared coping strategies, resources, and avenues for confidential reporting. Recognizing that systemic change required cultural change, we emphasized the importance of peer support and bystander intervention. I saw firsthand how hearing a survivor's truth could embolden others to come forward, dismantling the suffocating wall of silence piece by piece.

My outreach also extended into digital spaces where stigma and isolation often persisted. Managing social media accounts dedicated to MST awareness, I developed content that combined survivor stories, educational infographics, and live Q&A sessions with mental health professionals. These platforms became sanctuaries for survivors to connect across geographical distances, validating their experiences and fostering resilience. The immediacy and reach of online advocacy helped to demystify therapy, encourage disclosure, and direct survivors to vital support channels. However, I also encountered the inevitable backlash from trolls and skeptics, underscoring the persistent cultural resistance to confronting military sexual violence openly. Navigating this digital minefield demanded a thick skin and unwavering commitment to center the voices and needs of survivors above all else.

In parallel with grassroots efforts, I participated in shaping military training curricula by consulting on programs designed to educate service members about sexual harassment, assault prevention, and cultural competence. Drawing from my lived experience, I advocated fiercely for the inclusion of race-conscious approaches that acknowledged how racism intensified MST's impact on Black soldiers and how white supremacist factions within the military contributed to hostile environments. It was vital to expose these pernicious elements openly rather than treat MST as a gendered but otherwise homogeneous issue. Influencing such training was challenging; some military leaders resisted framing sexual assault through intersections of race and power, wary of opening old wounds or provoking institutional defensiveness. Yet, incremental progress was visible as diversity officers and new commanders increasingly recognized the need for honest dialogue about race, bias, and violence alongside sexual assault prevention.

Collaborations with mental health professionals deepened my advocacy's scope. Partnering with therapists specialized in trauma, substance abuse, and cultural competency allowed our campaigns to underscore the importance of timely intervention and comprehensive care. We worked to destigmatize therapy, especially for veterans of color who often mistrusted medical institutions due to historical abuses and systemic inequities. Public speaking engagements began to include testimonials from clinicians explaining treatments like Cognitive Processing Therapy (CPT) and pharmacological options and their critical role in recovery. Highlighting success stories and survivor resilience helped counter narratives of permanent victimhood, showing that with appropriate support, healing was possible even after the most grievous betrayals.

I also sought to honor the memories and struggles of others lost to MST-related despair—those who succumbed to addiction, homelessness, or suicide. During commemorative events and vigil ceremonies, I spoke solemnly of the hidden casualties of military sexual trauma, pressing for increased funding for mental health and housing assistance programs tailored for MST survivors. Bringing these human costs to light was an intimate yet vital part of advocacy, reminding audiences that prevention was not only about policy but about preserving human lives and rebuilding shattered souls.

As my visibility grew, so did invitations from mainstream media. I appeared in documentaries, podcasts, and interviews that reached audiences beyond veteran communities, amplifying MST's urgency in public consciousness. Media engagement was a double-edged sword—providing an expansive platform but also exposing me to scrutiny and the risk of re-traumatization. Navigating these encounters demanded careful boundary-setting, with a deliberate focus on educational messaging rather than sensationalism. Each appearance carried the potential to influence public opinion and political will, making the felt risk worthwhile.

Throughout this whirlwind of public engagement and outreach, I never lost sight of the core purpose: to transform pain into advocacy, isolation into solidarity, and silence into outcry. I carry the faces of those survivors I've met—the young recruit too ashamed to ask for help, the veteran struggling with addiction, the families fractured by trauma—reminding me that awareness is not an abstract ideal but a lifeline. Raising awareness is a daily act of courage and compassion, requiring persistent dedication amid setbacks and skepticism. It means holding space for survivors' truths, challenging outdated military cultures, and demanding accountability from institutions that have long failed us.

Ultimately, this advocacy work reshaped my own identity from victim to survivor, from broken to empowered. Speaking out publicly was more than a personal catharsis; it was a push against the tides of denial, a battle cry for justice and empathy, and a beacon to those still trapped in invisible chains. I now understand that breaking the silence about Military Sexual Trauma is not a finite destination but an ongoing, collective effort whose ripples can change lives, reform systems, and nurture hope. Through voice, visibility, and unyielding resolve, I stand to reclaim my story—not as a symbol of betrayal, but as a testament to resilience and the powerful force of raising awareness.

Policy Change

The call for policy change, especially within the realm of military sexual trauma and the Veterans Affairs system, was neither sudden nor easy. It was born from the deepest wells of pain and resilience, an intense intertwining of personal suffering and a fierce desire to protect others from the same desolation. Advocacy became a lifeline, a way to transform silence and shame into a potent force of reform and justice. Emerging from the shadow of trauma, the protagonist—once a hesitant, broken figure—found his voice growing stronger, more resolute, as he began to connect with organizations dedicated to the fight against military sexual assault and systemic failure. These organizations, often run by survivors and allies alike, provided not only community but strategic platforms to challenge longstanding institutional neglect and the deeply embedded culture that allowed MST to persist unchecked. Through public speaking engagements, written testimonies, and participation in survivor coalition meetings, he began to wield his experience not simply as a story of pain but as a weapon for change.

Within these networks, a vital intersection of voices converged—survivors from all ranks, advocacy groups, mental health professionals, and sympathetic lawmakers—each driven by a shared urgency to overhaul the military's approach toward prevention, accountability, and support. The weight of the protagonist's narrative lent urgency to these efforts, demonstrating viscerally how racism and violence intertwined within the military hierarchy and how VA resources, while a potential sanctuary, were often mired in bureaucracy and old stigmas. He became intimately involved in campaigns that called for mandatory training on sexual violence prevention that included cultural competency and anti-racist frameworks. More than rote compliance, these initiatives insisted on a fundamental shift in military culture—the kind of cultural re-education that could erode the breeding ground of prejudice and impunity. By collaborating with experts in legal reform, he advocated for stronger punitive measures against assault perpetrators, pushing to dismantle existing whistle-blower retaliation laws that often silenced victims. The goal was clear: to create an environment where truth was honored and safety not just promised but guaranteed.

His grassroots activism often brought him face to face with veterans struggling silently within the VA system, a bureaucracy chronically fraught with underfunding, understaffing, and, at times, a pervasive skepticism toward claims of MST. These encounters reiterated the critical need for reform—not just at the legislative level but also in how VA facilities operated daily. The focus shifted to improving screening procedures, making trauma-informed care accessible outside large urban centers, and ensuring the inclusion of therapist training on race and sexual trauma's unique interactions. The protagonist championed the expansion of Cognitive Processing Therapy (CPT) efficacy studies and better integration of medication-assisted treatments, emphasizing how healing must be tailored, holistic, and recognized as a complex, ongoing journey rather than a quick fix. Through policy forums and closed-door meetings with VA officials, his lived experience became a case study demanding systemic recalibration. It was a painstaking process, rife with bureaucratic inertia and resistance from old-guard officials who feared exposing institutional flaws, but inch by inch, progress was made.

One of the pivotal steps in his advocacy was helping to draft and promote legislation aimed at providing clearer pathways for MST survivors to claim benefits without facing the torment of repeated victimization through endless paperwork or hostile interrogations. The laws he pushed for sought to streamline access to mental health services while protecting survivors from the retaliation that had long been a silent norm. He also advocated for the establishment of survivor advisory boards within the military and VA structures, ensuring that those most affected had direct input into shaping policies that affect their lives. This component was vital. It rejected the old model where experts and policymakers spoke on behalf of survivors; instead, survivors were recognized as indispensable agents of change, their insights fundamental to any real reform. The protagonist took part in public hearings and congressional briefings, where his testimony often moved lawmakers beyond statistics to a palpable human reality, convincing many that ignoring MST was not just morally indefensible but politically untenable.

Equally significant was his work to bring racial dynamics into sharper focus in the national conversation about MST. While the military had long touted diversity and inclusion, the persistent presence of white supremacist groups within its ranks underscored the urgent need to confront the systemic racism enabling assault and intimidation. The protagonist's story was a stark repudiation of any sanitized narratives, forcing policymakers to grapple with the ways in which racial violence and sexual trauma were intertwined and inseparable from military service for many Black soldiers. He worked closely with civil rights organizations to embed stronger anti-racist measures into military training and accountability procedures. His advocacy extended to demanding increased transparency about hate group activity in the armed forces and the creation of specialized investigative units within the military police tasked with rooting out racially motivated abuse. By linking race and MST explicitly in reform efforts, he helped expand the scope of survivor protections and education programs—moving the issue from being seen solely as a "women's issue" to a broader, more inclusive understanding of intersectional violence. This fueled a renewed commitment among policymakers and military leaders to prioritize the dismantling of hate networks that permeated the very institutions sworn to defend.

As a survivor who had walked the treacherous path from victimization to empowerment, the protagonist's personal evolution was inseparable from his advocacy. His willingness to publicly share his story broke longstanding taboos and challenged the entrenched stoicism within veteran communities. Speaking engagements at universities, military bases, and national conventions not only educated but inspired others to come forward, creating a ripple effect of awareness and solidarity. The authenticity of his voice shattered the myth of invulnerability often imposed on service members, revealing vulnerability as strength and healing as a collective responsibility. His participation in media interviews and documentary projects further amplified the call for reform, reaching audiences who may never have confronted MST otherwise. Each narrative chapter he added to public discourse chipped away at stigma, fostering spaces where survivors could find validation and access resources. His advocacy underscored the idea that acknowledging pain was not weakness but a crucial first step toward institutional transformation and personal redemption.

Collaboration became a cornerstone of his efforts as he bridged gaps among diverse groups—connecting survivors across gender lines, racial backgrounds, and military branches to form coalitions with unified voices. These alliances were instrumental in lobbying Congress to appropriate increased funding for MST programs and research, and they pushed the Department of Defense to revise investigative protocols that too often left victims without justice. Within these spaces, the protagonist also emphasized the importance of survivor self-care and peer support initiatives, arguing that policy must not only address external systems but nurture internal community healing. He supported the development of mentorship programs pairing newly discharged veterans with survivors who are further along in their recovery, fostering resilience and a sense of belonging. Policy reform, he insisted, had to move beyond punitive measures and clinical treatments to embrace holistic wellness and empowerment. This comprehensive approach helped expand funding streams and ensured that new regulations translated into practical, accessible, and effective support on the ground.

Perhaps most transformative was his involvement in pushing for changes that recognized the long-term nature of MST's impact. Traditional policies often set rigid time limits or narrow criteria for accessing benefits or treatment, ignoring how survivors' needs evolve over years or even decades. The protagonist advocated for the removal of these arbitrary barriers and for the institutional acknowledgment of the chronic mental health challenges stemming from MST, including PTSD, depression, and substance use disorders. His work helped spur legislative amendments allowing for lifetime eligibility for MST-related care and fostering a continuum of support that adapted to survivors' changing circumstances. He also fought for better tracking and data collection within the military and VA so that policymakers could tailor interventions based on real-time evidence rather than outdated assumptions. Such data-driven reforms promised more efficient resource allocation and meaningful outcome measurement—tools essential for sustaining progress and preventing future generations of service members from languishing in neglect.

This intense dedication to policy advocacy was not without its emotional costs. The protagonist often revisited his trauma during testimony sessions and strategy meetings, each recounting a double-edged sword—painful yet empowering. The re-exposure tested his resilience but also deepened his conviction that system change was a moral imperative. By transforming personal agony into collective action, he embodied the paradox of healing through activism. His efforts illuminated the realities of survivors often obscured by institutional silence, turning their stories into powerful instruments of accountability and hope. His legacy took root in new military directives promoting transparency, victim-centered investigations, and mandatory reporting reforms designed to dismantle the culture of silence that had sheltered perpetrators for too long. At the VA level, his contributions shaped enhanced training protocols and expanded access to trauma-informed care, ensuring that survivors encountered understanding and respect rather than distrust or dismissal.

Ultimately, his advocacy reframed the national narrative about military service, acknowledging the complexities of honor and betrayal, courage and victimization. By championing comprehensive reforms that addressed the vicious cycle of racial violence, sexual trauma, and institutional neglect, he helped forge a path toward a military and veteran system rooted in integrity, justice, and healing. His journey from a broken teenager seeking escape to a fearless advocate demanding transformation serves as a testament to the power of voice and the indispensability of systemic change. Through relentless commitment and strategic alliances, he transformed his story into a beacon for others to dare to hope, speak out, and reclaim their futures. This labor of advocacy, both deeply personal and powerfully political, ensured that no survivor would face the shadow alone or unheard, bringing the promise of a future where betrayal could give way to trust restored and lives rebuilt.